Pediatric Surgical Procedures - An Updated Guide - Volume 2

Edited by Sherif Shehata

Published in London, United Kingdom

Pediatric Surgical Procedures - An Updated Guide - Volume 2
http://dx.doi.org/10.5772/intechopen.1008022
Edited by Sherif Shehata

Contributors
Aidan Weitzner, Alison Ford Martinez de Pinillos, Aruna Kumar Dash, Ayush Kumar Dash, Chad Crigger, Elena Țarcă, Ilhama Jafarli, Jason Yang, Luis Fernando Monasterio Roman, Luis Monasterio Aljaro, Melissa A. LoPresti, Nitisha Narayan, Pramod Kumar Mohanty, Ryan Kelly, Samar Mousa, Sandi Lam

First published in London, United Kingdom, 2026 by IntechOpen
IntechOpen is the global imprint of INTECHOPEN LIMITED, registered in England and Wales, registration number: 11086078, 167-169 Great Portland Street, London, W1W 5PF, United Kingdom

For EU product safety concerns: IN TECH d.o.o., Prolaz Marije Krucifikse Kozulić 3, 51000 Rijeka, Croatia, info@intechopen.com or visit our website at intechopen.com.

British Library Cataloguing-in-Publication Data
A catalogue record for this book is available from the British Library

Pediatric Surgical Procedures - An Updated Guide - Volume 2
Edited by Sherif Shehata
p. cm.
Print ISBN 978-1-83635-199-3
Online ISBN 978-1-83635-198-6
eBook (PDF) ISBN 978-1-83635-200-6

If disposing of this product, please recycle the paper responsibly.

Meet the editor

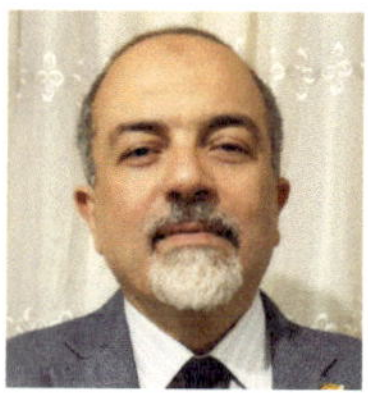

Dr. Sherif Shehata was born in Egypt in 1965. He graduated from Tanta Medical School in 1988 with honors; then he began his residency at Tanta University Hospital and Abo Elreesh Children's Hospital in Cairo. He got his master's in surgery in 1993; then he received a grant to pursue his Ph.D. He trained at Sophia Children's Hospital, Rotterdam, Netherlands (1996–2000), and at Alder Hey Children's Hospital, Liverpool, UK (1998). He got his Ph.D. from Erasmus University in Rotterdam in November 1999. He completed specialty training in the Netherlands. He received an MD (Surg) from Tanta University in 2001. He has been a Full Professor of Pediatric Surgery since 2011. He was the former vice dean of postgraduate studies and research at the Medical Faculty in Tanta, Egypt (2015–2018) and EPSA president (2020–2021). Since 2001, he has been a Professor and Chief of Pediatric Surgery at Tanta University, Egypt. He is also the President of the Egyptian Promotion Committee for Professorship in Pediatric Surgery, Supreme Council of the Egyptian Universities (2022 - 2025); President of IPEG–MEC (International Pediatric Endosurgery Group- Middle East Chapter) (since 2023), and a member of the Higher Committee of CPD in the Egyptian Health Council (since 2023). Over the last fifteen years, he has dedicated a significant portion of his time and effort to training junior pediatric surgeons, especially in MIS, Laparoscopy, and pediatric urology. He conducts workshops in various countries across the Middle East, including Egypt, Libya, Tunisia, Algeria, Morocco, Turkey, Iraq, Saudi Arabia, Kuwait, Uzbekistan, Italy, Chile, the UK, and Portugal. He has over 82 publications, including 51 international peer-reviewed journal articles and four book chapters. He participated in more than 310 conferences and workshops with more than 193 presentations.

Contents

Preface

Surgical procedures are always tailored to achieve the best possible outcome for the patient. This point is of utmost importance and interest, from the oldest known civilization (Pharaonic Egypt) to now, especially for our kids.

Junior Pediatric Surgeons are treated humbly by their seniors in training, as they will take care of the future community.

The need for young pediatric surgeons to update their knowledge, which will be reflected in pediatric care, was the ambition behind this series. As the surgical art has no limits, we aim to simplify surgical knowledge and skills in an appealing way across different disciplines. We aim to update theoretical information, clinical decision-making, and surgical steps through chapters with numerous illustrations and figures that guide the surgeon's decisions and support competent training and skill development.

In the current second volume of this book, seven chapters are included, starting with a neonatal section covering two common neonatal pathologies: gastroschisis and pyloric stenosis (IHPS) that need urgent interventions. Then, Section 2 presents two major reconstructive procedures: a unique collection of rare median cleft lip cases with more than 30 figures, followed by cleft palate management from another perspective.

Section 3, covering pediatric urology in two chapters, provides updated knowledge on androgen insensitivity syndrome and DSD, with a stepwise management approach, followed by an updated robotic pyeloplasty. The final chapter in this volume presents the concept of functional surgery in a very special and common situation, with the most recent treatment from a leading center in this field, although it is not within the scope of general pediatric surgery practice.

I consider this second volume a further step toward achieving our goals by providing science and education for every pediatric surgeon and, hopefully, whetting readers' appetites for future volumes. In this updated guide to pediatric surgery procedures, we hope to help all pediatric surgeons, whether residents or specialists, improve their practice across the broad field of pediatric surgery.

I appreciate all authors, co-authors, and contributors who, without their effort, this final version of the book could not have been completed.

Dr. Sherif Shehata, MB.BCh, M.Ch, CST, Ph.D., M.D (Surg)
Professor,
Professor of Pediatric Surgery,
Pediatric Surgery Section,
Tanta Faculty of Medicine,
Tanta, Egypt

Section 1

Neonatal Surgery

Chapter 1

Gastroschisis Management

Elena Țarcă

Abstract

Congenital defects of the anterior abdominal wall (celosomies) are among the most common congenital malformations and are represented by omphalocele, gastroschisis, bladder exstrophy, cloacal exstrophy, and prune-belly syndrome. Omphalocele and gastroschisis are the most common types of congenital defects of the anterior abdominal wall. This chapter describes the main gastroschisis characteristics regarding prenatal, obstetric, and postnatal management, and also its etiopathogenesis, clinical appearance, malformative associations, and prognosis. The main purpose of this chapter is to describe the technique for reducing the viscera in the peritoneal cavity and closing the anterior abdominal wall defect primarily when possible, or with the help of prosthetic materials in case of viscero-abdominal disproportion. Even though opinions on the best time and method of delivery are divided, prompt medical and surgical treatment in a tertiary neonatal critical care unit can guarantee a survival rate of more than 90% in cases of gastroschisis.

Keywords: abdominal wall defects, neonate, gastroschisis, abdominal compartment syndrome, silo-bag

1. Introduction

Human civilization has always placed a high value on medicine, and congenital malformations have long been a source of concern. In the majority of the world's nations, congenital abnormalities are still a major cause of infant morbidity and mortality, and the prevalence of malformations appears to be rising despite advancements in biomedical science. The earliest written mentions of intestinal and genital deformities date to 2000 BC and are found on Chaldean cuneiform tablets. Gastroschisis was first reported in detail by James Calder of Glasgow in 1733. Fear performed the first primary closure operation on a patient with gastroschisis in 1878, but the patient did not survive. In his essay "Anatomical Philosophy - Human Monstrosity" from 1832, Etienne Geoffroy Saint-Hilaire provides a thorough description of anterior abdominal wall abnormalities. The appearance of intestinal loops in gastroschisis cases was meticulously described by Bernstein in 1940, who noted "the absence of a covering membrane leading to significant dilatation and thickening of the intestinal wall, with cyanosis and adhesion of the loops, in fact the evisceration usually presenting itself as a solid mass containing agglutinated intestinal loops." Reed reported a case of successfully operated gastroschisis in 1913 [1, 2]. Moore and Stokes first brought attention to the confusion between omphalocele and gastroschisis in 1953, arguing that these were two distinct conditions. In that study, the clinical aspects of these abnormalities were precisely documented, and the thickening of intestinal loops in gastroschisis was named "chemical peritonitis." Additionally, they classified "congenital eviscerations of the anterior abdominal wall" in a clinical manner for the first time [3]. Despite being a relatively benign malformation, gastroschisis is associated with significant neonatal morbidity, and there is still disagreement regarding the best way to deliver it, when to do it, how to treat it, and the main risk factors for morbidities [4].

2. Natural history aspects in gastroschisis

Although there is debate on the etiopathogenesis of this abdominal abnormality, the majority of physicians concur that it is caused by a vascular accident that involves the right omphalo-mesenteric artery [5], though a small percentage of instances may be the consequence of an omphalocele rupture that occurs during pregnancy [6]. The fact that mothers who take vasopressor drugs during pregnancy, such as cocaine, nicotine, and pseudoephedrine, have a higher prevalence of gastroschisis supports vascular theories. It has been demonstrated that maternal vascular hypoperfusion, as evidenced by placental analysis, causes intermittent fetal ischemia, resulting in intrauterine growth restriction of the fetus and placenta as well as abnormalities at the cerebral, myocardial, and anterior abdominal wall [7]. The entire digestive tract usually eviscerates and floats freely in the amniotic fluid in the absence of an encasing sac. The intestines' shorter length, thicker mesentery, and the formation of a thick inflammatory barrier on their surface are all linked to decreased motility and nutrient absorption (**Figure 1**).

Kiesewetter initially described the so-called closed gastroschisis in 1957; in this condition, the abdominal wall defect (AWD) closes around the eviscerated intestinal loop, causing the loop to necrotize and vanish in utero [8]. From modest adhesions between the intestinal loops and the tiny parietal defect to the "vanishing midgut," where the intestine vanished due to necrosis and intrauterine resorption, there have been numerous cases documented in the literature (**Figure 2**). The anterior AWD then fully closes, giving the umbilical area an almost normal appearance.

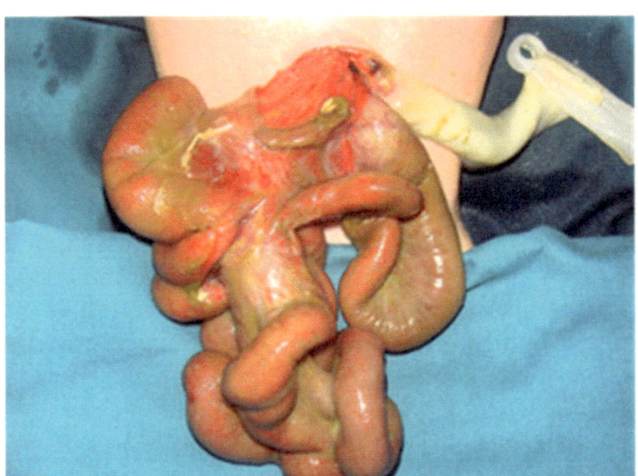

Figure 1.
Thick inflammatory membrane covering intestinal loops in gastroschisis, making peristalsis inefficient in the first weeks of life.

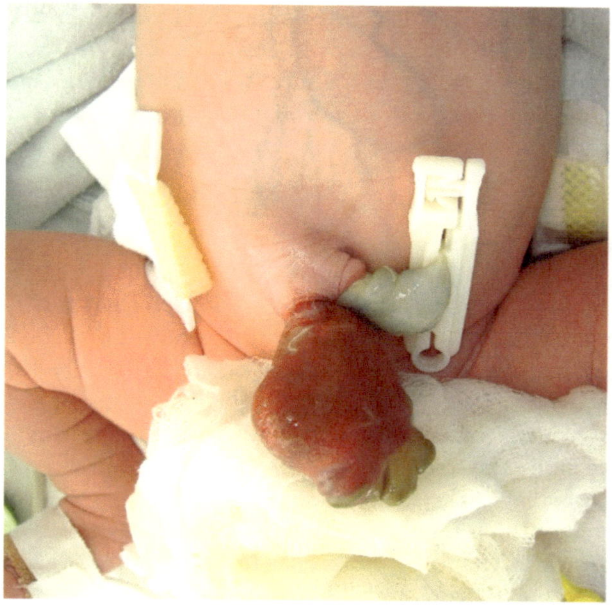

Figure 2.
Vanishing (complex) gastroschisis, meaning intrauterine resorptions of eviscerated loops.

Occasionally, the eviscerated intestinal loops are neither edematous nor substantially altered at birth, nor are they covered by that inflammatory membrane; venous blockage and protein transudate, which dries at room temperature, cause these alterations after birth (**Figure 3**). Since the intestinal wall seems normal at birth in many situations, it is unclear if the amniotic fluid is the cause of those alterations. Consequently, some writers dispute the justification for premature birth, particularly in light of other authors' findings that patients with gastroschisis born at term have a superior prognosis [9].

In 2001, Molik proposed a straightforward yet useful distinction between simple and complex gastroschisis based on the intestinal abnormalities and prognosis [10].

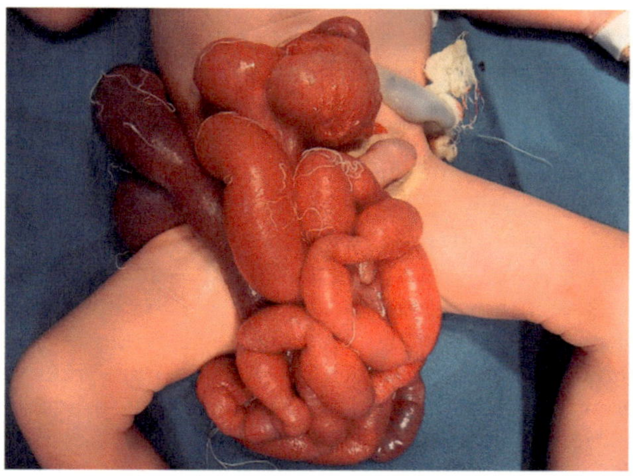

Figure 3.
Almost normal appearance of intestinal loops at birth in gastroschisis.

Intestinal atresia and stenosis, which can be simple or multiple levels (most are type 3a), are associated with gastroschisis in 5–25% of instances. These conditions can result in substantial morbidity and a 40% mortality rate. Necrosis of eviscerated loops or their perforation may occur in 4–5% of cases, as a result of atresia with overlying distension, volvulus, or chemical peritonitis [11].

3. Epidemiological aspects

Globally, the incidence and prevalence of anterior AWDs—particularly gastroschisis (also called laparoschisis)—have increased in recent years, according to published research, the incidence of gastroschisis varying between 0.5–5.99/10,000 newborns in Europe [12, 13]. For the first time in decades, the prevalence of gastroschisis in the US is declining, according to three extensive national datasets from 2016 to 2022 [14]. Some studies have demonstrated an equal gender distribution of gastroschisis, while others have shown a small male predominance with a high of 1.68 [15]. The disadvantaged maternal population is more likely to have congenital defects of the abdominal wall, according to studies that consider socioeconomic factors. This is likely due to low maternal age, frequent drugs and medication used during pregnancy, smoking, lack of family planning in this population, and unmarried status [16]. The occurrence of some congenital malformations can be significantly influenced by the environment. For example, pollution from large, highly industrialized urban agglomerations has increased the incidence of gastroschisis or cleft palate in some cities in Finland, the USA, the UK, and Poland [17]. Chemicals used in agriculture and present in drinking water, such as atrazine, arsenic, or nitrates, can cause teratogenic effects during pregnancy. These consequences include limb abnormalities, neural tube defects, AWDs, and other congenital malformations [18, 19].

4. Antenatal diagnostic

Nowadays, ultrasound of the pregnant uterus may detect gastroschisis antenatally in 18–100% of cases because of advancements in ultrasound instrument resolution and the expertise of specialized physicians [20]. An extra-abdominal "cystic mass" (eviscerated, dilated, fluid-filled intestinal loops) floating freely in excess amniotic fluid was Grossman's first description of the sonographic look of gastroschisis in 1978 [21]. The earliest gastroschisis diagnosis is made at 12 weeks, and it is most frequently made between 16 and 24 weeks of amenorrhea (mean 20 weeks). A 2–4 cm diameter defect in the right paramedian anterior abdominal wall, next to the distinct and normal insertion of the umbilical cord, may be seen on sonography, supporting the diagnosis of gastroschisis (**Figure 4**). The abdominal viscera—typically the intestinal loops, but less frequently the stomach or other organs—are externalized through this hole and lack a membrane covering. Although the liver is normally found intra-abdominally, gastroschisis with an eviscerated liver is a rare occurrence. The evisceration of the abdominal organs also results in a reduction of the transverse diameter and the circumference of the abdominal cavity. Unfavorable prognostic variables for postnatal evolution include intestinal loop dilatation and intestinal wall thickening. Excellent visualization of the umbilical vessel course and precise separation of eviscerated intestinal loops from the umbilical cord—which can be mistaken for the former—are made possible by color Doppler ultrasonography.

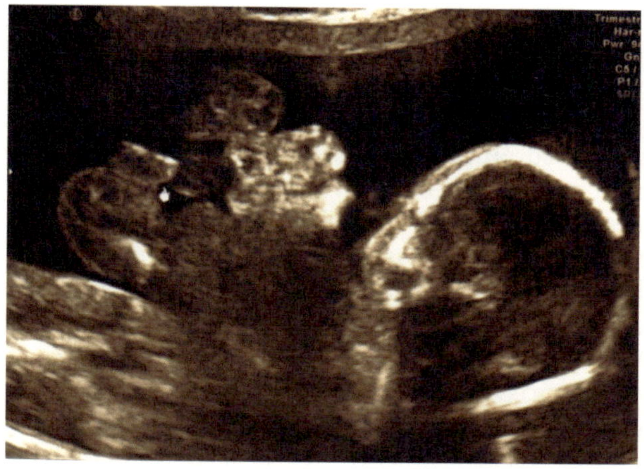

Figure 4.
Antenatal diagnosis of gastroschisis—18 gestational weeks, showing eviscerated loops besides the umbilical cord.

Three-dimensional ultrasound is used in addition to traditional ultrasound to diagnose and assess fetuses with abnormalities of the abdominal wall. In any situation where there are diagnostic challenges or related abnormalities, the combination of the two methods is advised. The intestinal loops, liver, and spleen are seen on fetal MRI, but it is more challenging to distinguish between the small and large intestine because meconium builds up in the large intestine toward the end of pregnancy. Fetal MRI exams can essentially determine the presence, location, and extent of anterior AWD. They should only be used in conjunction with ultrasound exams in specific situations where more data is required to decide whether to terminate a pregnancy therapeutically or to plan postnatal therapeutic management. For instance, according to a 2021 study, fetal MRI can predict silo-bag treatment in 90% of cases for patients with gastroschisis [22].

The presence of an anterior AWD, such as gastroschisis, limb body wall complex, or bladder or cloacal exstrophy, may also be indicated by a rise in maternal serum and in amniotic fluid alpha-fetoprotein during the second trimester of pregnancy, because this marker is not a particular indicator of neurological abnormalities. Amniotic fluid can be used to assess acetylcholinesterase, which seems to be elevated in cases of fetal neural tube abnormalities, ruptured omphalocele, gastroschisis, and cloacal exstrophy.

5. Prenatal management

Even though fetuses with gastroschisis have a high survival rate, the length of hospitalization and the expense of surgical therapy for these patients are significant. This is because prolonged exposure of the intestinal loops to the irritating action of amniotic fluid causes the intestinal wall to thicken and fibrin deposits to develop, which negatively impact peristalsis and transit resumption. Although the findings of many studies have been conflicting, amniotic fluid exchange or amnioinfusion can minimize the adverse consequences of amniotic fluid exposure and oligohydramnios by reducing the quantity of dangerous chemicals [23]. It is necessary to weigh the potential for major problems and adverse effects against the improvement of intestinal lesions from plastic peritonitis in gastroschisis following amniotic exchanges or amnioinfusion.

The effects of some substances administered through amniotic puncture have recently drawn experimental attention. These substances may have a trophic effect on the intestinal mucosa, increasing its absorption capacity, or reduce peritonitis phenomena at the level of eviscerated intestinal loops. These effects could contribute to efficient postnatal absorption and peristalsis, a quicker start to enteral nutrition, and, implicitly, a shorter hospital stay and cost. The effects of intra-amniotic administration of stem cells, recombinant human erythropoietin, sodium bicarbonate, furosemide, nitric oxide, and corticosteroid or other anti-inflammatories have been investigated in this context [24–26].

In the instance of human gastroschisis, the hazards of fetal surgery—specifically, the possibility of problems that could result in an early birth—now exceed the advantages of in utero surgical intervention [23].

Late in pregnancy, spontaneous abortion in gastroschisis frequently occurs. It may be brought on by a vagal response, gastric or intestinal perforation, tension on the mesentery, abrupt dilatation of the intestinal loops, and compression of the umbilical cord and umbilical vessels [20, 27]. Because the deformity is deemed incompatible with life, therapeutic abortion is recommended in cases of malformative associations, such as the limb body wall complex, which can be identified by ultrasound as early as the first trimester of pregnancy.

6. Fetal monitoring and birth scheduling

Following the prenatal diagnosis, the family receives appropriate counseling, the birth is planned in terms of time, type, and location, and the medical staff is ready to step in as soon as possible and as suitably as possible, starting from the very first minutes of extrauterine life. A skilled obstetric team must assist in the delivery of a child with an AWD in a level three hospital unit. A team of pediatric surgeons with specialized training must then transport the newborn to an intensive care unit and neonatal resuscitation unit, where they must have access to a modern operating room. Without significantly increasing morbidity from prematurity, scheduled preterm delivery at 36–37 weeks gestational age, based on preestablished ultrasound parameters, has improved postoperative prognosis. However, other research supports the better prognosis of children born at term by highlighting the drawbacks of prematurity, particularly when combined with a deficient neonatal intensive care unit [9, 28].

Given the controversy over routine cesarean sections for children with congenital anterior abdominal wall abnormalities, the mode of delivery should be based solely on obstetric considerations. Since there are no statistically significant differences in the risk of per primam parietal closure, neonatal sepsis, mortality, time to cessation of total parenteral nutrition, or hospitalization period, the meta-analysis of the specialized literature on the delivery of children with gastroschisis does not emphasize the superiority of systematic delivery by cesarean section [29].

7. Pre-operative medical therapeutic management

With the medical staff ready to take over under ideal circumstances, the newborn with an AWD identified prenatally will be born in a specialized facility, improving the prognosis. For a comprehensive evaluation to be conducted in the delivery room, a neonatologist must be present. It is necessary to clamp and cut the umbilical cord far enough from the abdominal wall to prevent intestinal loop injury. If the cord is left long, it can be used as autologous material to cover the wall defect in gastroschisis. Examining the intestinal loops to make sure they are not twisted is necessary to ensure there is an adequate circulatory supply. An excessively narrow parietal ring should not compress the mesentery. The AWD should be enlarged right away if it is too small and results in ischemia in the disemboweled organs. The next step is a comprehensive physical examination that includes a rectal examination, a nasogastric tube pass for abdominal decompression, meconium elimination stimulation, and the detection of any related digestive disorders. An immediate venous line and a urethrovesical catheter will be inserted. In addition to receiving fluids, vitamin K, and antibiotic prophylaxis, the infant will be placed in the incubator in the right lateral decubitus position, and biological samples will be taken for routine analysis.

Until the moment of operation, the abdominal viscera should be kept in a sterile, non-adherent, waterproof bag. The safest period to operate for gastroschisis, according to cardiology, is within the first 15 minutes of delivery, when right ventricular compliance has not yet decreased and a left-to-right shunt has not yet developed as a result of a septal defect or patent ductus arteriosus. Furthermore, the less edematous the intestinal loops are at the time of surgery, the higher the likelihood of primary closure, and the lower the risk of intestinal dysfunction [30].

8. Integration of viscera into the peritoneal cavity and primary closure of the abdominal wall defect

After being taken to the operating room, the newborn will have a bladder catheter inserted to track diuresis and a central venous catheter placed. After swabbing the belly and perineum with an aqueous chlorhexidine solution to prepare the surgical field, the extra umbilical cord will be cut off. Maintaining a proper body temperature throughout the surgical procedure is crucial; to do this, sticky fields and blankets can be utilized to reduce heat loss. Integrating the intestinal loops into the abdomen and closing the fascia are the objectives of surgical treatment; in many cases, this is achievable per primam.

The patient is intubated, sedatives are administered, and morphine is used for intraoperative and postoperative pain management. Curarization is an option if preventing abdominal hypertension requires improved muscular relaxation. High-frequency oscillatory ventilation may be employed in cases of respiratory distress or pulmonary hypoplasia, although mechanical ventilation will be the standard treatment for the majority of patients. After disinfecting the skin, the externalized viscera's volume and appearance are examined. The intestinal loops will be gently introduced into the belly by taxis if the conditions are suitable (no serious lesions of plastic peritonitis, atresia, or perforations) and the parietal defect is not too narrow (**Figure 5**). A 2–3 cm supraumbilical median incision can be used to widen a parietal defect that is too narrow. This is preferable to a transverse incision, which is unattractive and increases the risk of ventral hernias. The abdominal wall will be closed in three planes using distinct sutures, either longitudinally or transversely, if this can be done without causing an unacceptable rise in abdominal pressure (**Figure 6**).

Bianchi and Dickson introduced "minimal intervention management," which refers to integrating intestinal loops through the parietal defect in the neonatal intensive care unit or even in the incubator without the use of sedatives or general anesthesia, at approximately 4 hours after birth, when the newborn becomes cardiocirculatory and respiratory stable [31].

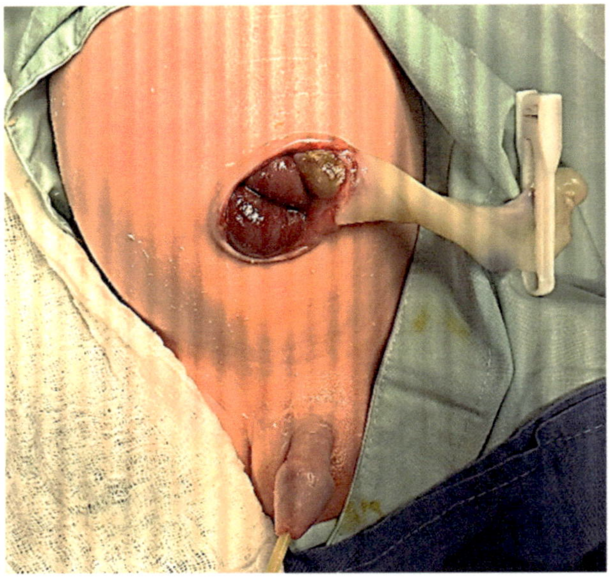

Figure 5.
Complete integration of viscera into the peritoneal cavity.

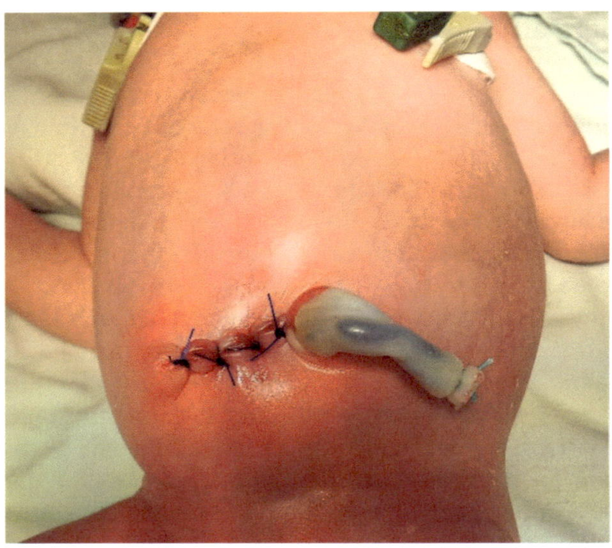

Figure 6.
Per primam closure of the AWD in a transverse manner.

Sandler and associates suggest "plastic" closure of the gastroschisis, which involves integrating the intestinal loops into the peritoneal cavity with or without general anesthesia. However, the abdominal wall will not be sealed under tension; instead, it will be covered with the umbilical cord, which will be cut lengthwise and constructed in accordance with the defect's dimensions [32]. At this level, granulation tissue appears, which will later be epithelialized. The benefit of using the umbilical cord in this manner is that the patient and surgeon can access it right away, and the rate of complications seems to be lower (**Figure** 7).

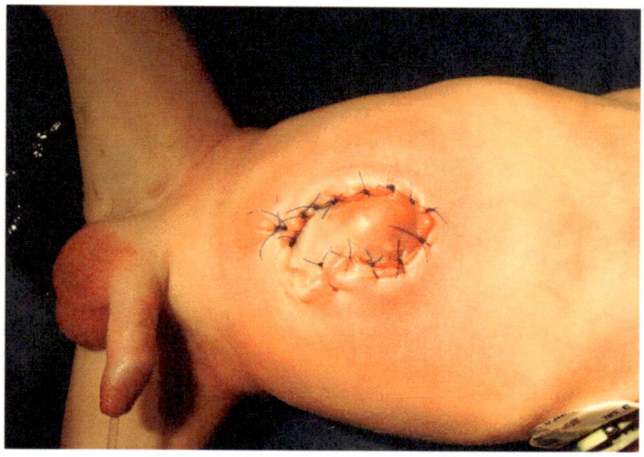

Figure 7.
Umbilical cord patch for expanding the surface of the abdominal wall.

The best way to handle complex gastroschisis situations is still up for debate in the literature. Rather than the treatment technique (per primam/per secundam ileostomy or resection and primary anastomosis), the variations in the outcomes following the implementation of different management strategies are a reflection of the location of the atresia, the degree of intestinal loop involvement, and the heterogeneity of the circumstances of individuals with gastroschisis. Therefore, based on each patient's unique clinical situation, different management techniques should be used [33].

9. Abdominal compartment syndrome

The small and underdeveloped peritoneal cavity may press on the contents of the abdomen, cause ventilatory problems, compress the inferior vena cava and mesenteric veins, hamper hepatic and renal circulation, and have a lack of venous return. Monitoring intragastric or intravesical pressure, comparing peripheral oxygenation at the level of the upper and lower limbs (the difference that must not exceed 10%), and monitoring respiratory constants are all necessary to identify these alterations early, during surgery, and after. A newborn's normal abdominal pressure ranges from 1 to 8 mm Hg; if it is higher than 15 mm Hg, it is referred to as abdominal hyper-pressure; if it is higher than 20 mm Hg, there is a high chance of developing *abdominal compartment syndrome*, which can have major hemodynamic and respiratory repercussions [34]. Intraoperative measurement of abdominal pressure to avoid abdominal compartment syndrome can be done simply with the help of a urinary catheter connected to a manometer. Saline is introduced onto the urinary catheter to fill the urinary bladder with 1 ml/kg of body weight. The pressure is measured 30–60 seconds after instillation, at the end of expiration, taking the iliac crest (zero point) as a reference. According to Olesevich's study, intraoperative measurement of bladder pressure improves the safety of primary closure, avoids ischemia of intestinal loops, and shortens the time to enteral nutrition initiation as well as the total length of hospital stay [35].

Another method for early detection of abdominal compartment syndrome is gastric tonometry, which measures the CO_2 concentration in the gastric mucosa, which is higher in cases of decreased tissue perfusion [36].

From a hemodynamic perspective, abdominal compartment syndrome decreases cardiac output by lowering venous return, produces arterial hypotension, and, secondarily, results in intestinal and renal ischemia. Drug metabolism is also affected by oligo-anuria, intestinal mucosal acidosis, hypoventilation, and changes in hepatic venous flow.

10. Abdominal wall defect closure by the Schuster method

A temporary bag of inextensible synthetic material will be used to gradually integrate the herniated viscera over 1–14 days if their introduction into the peritoneal cavity is not possible without causing a marked increase in intra-abdominal pressure and the hazards that go along with it. Schuster originally introduced this technique in 1967, and it can be used for both big omphaloceles and gastroschisis [37]. This method was refined in 1969 by Allen and Wrenn, who used a single Dacron plate that was suspended from the incubator's roof by a traction wire after being sutured circularly across the AWD [38]. Consequently, under their weight, the viscera were able to progressively and fully integrate into the peritoneal cavity. Teflon plates were gradually replaced by simple or prefabricated Silastic plates, Gore-Tex, Prolene, or polypropylene plates, or other high-quality prosthetic materials over time [39]. In their absence, PVC bags used for blood transfusions or other sterile inert materials were successfully used (**Figure 8**).

10.1 Preloaded silo method

Preformed silastic bags, also known as "silo-bags," come in a variety of sizes and are used most frequently these days. They have a harder ring at the base and are placed beneath the edges of the AWD. The intestinal loops are then inserted inside

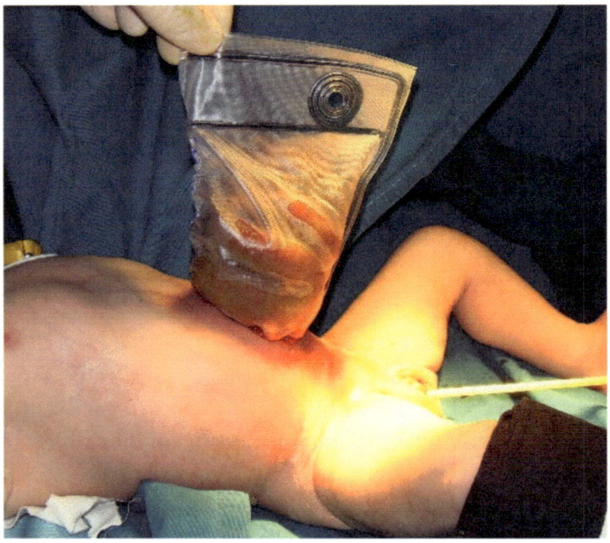

Figure 8.
Sterile urinary PVC bag used for gradually integrating intestinal loops into the peritoneal cavity.

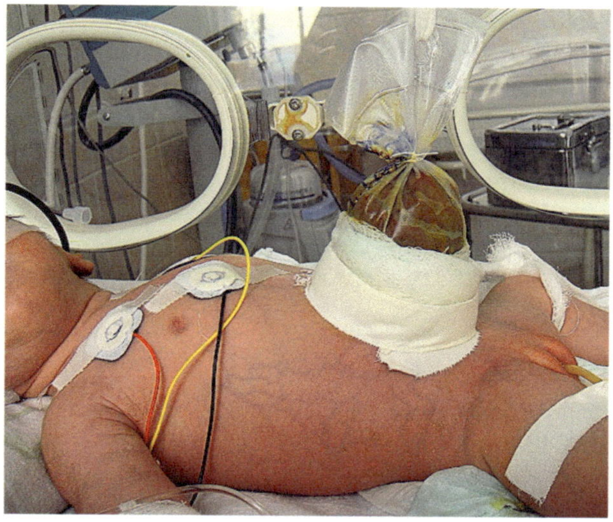

Figure 9.
Ligation of the silo-bag from the tip to the base, for progressive integration of the intestinal loops.

the bag, sometimes with general anesthesia and other times without, only under light sedation and at the patient's bedside [40]. Since infection is the method's most dreaded risk, the wound edges are cleaned every day and securely bandaged with antibiotic ointment [41]. The loops are introduced into the belly gradually over 1 to 14 days by progressively clamping or ligating the plastic bag from the tip to the base once a day (**Figure 9**). After the fascia has been closed, the abdominal wall is definitively closed in the operating room by forming two skin flaps that are sutured horizontally.

Numerous studies examine how the outcomes of primary closure differ from those of the "silo" strategy; the majority of retrospective studies report improved outcomes following primary closure [42]. However, recent research indicates that patients treated using the "silo" method require fewer days of mechanical ventilation, but there are no appreciable variations in the duration of parenteral nutrition or the transition to total enteral feeding. While the "silo" method is linked to a shorter duration of mechanical ventilation and lower ventilatory pressures, with fewer days of hospitalization, lower overall costs, and a lower rate of complications, primary closure is linked to the need for mechanical ventilation at higher pressures, an increased need for oxygen and vasopressors, and a risk of acute renal failure [43–45]. However, in order to give the criteria required for determining the best therapy choice, prospective studies involving larger patient groups are required.

11. Alternative methods for closing the abdominal wall defect

11.1 Abdominal wall defect closure by the Gross method

Gross described in 1948 (adapted by Moore in 1953) a method of delayed integration of the abdominal viscera into the peritoneal cavity, to avoid a sudden increase in intra-abdominal pressure: initially, the viscera are introduced into the abdomen without pressure, and the wall defect is covered with skin flaps advanced from the side [3, 46]. The result is a residual ventral hernia that will be treated secondarily after 6–18 months. The original Gross method has some disadvantages, such as ignoring possible associated digestive malformations, significant detachment of the skin with associated infectious risk and unsatisfactory cosmetic result, and last but not least, the need for surgical reintervention to resolve the remaining hernia and muscle dehiscence. This procedure is now only used in conjunction with other methods, such as parietal closure with an inert synthetic plate placed between the margins of the rectus abdominis muscles, due to the risk of bleeding, infection, and skin necrosis. The created skin flaps cover the synthetic plate, which in turn covers and shields the abdominal viscera.

11.2 New alternative methods of closure

As new technological advancements in medical bioengineering emerged, contemporary biocompatible materials that do not cling to the underlying visceral mass and permit the formation of granulation tissue on top started to be used in surgery. Over time, a variety of synthetic materials—including Teflon, Dacron, Gore-Tex, Marlex, Vicryl, and Silastic—of progressively greater quality have been used. Some authors have also effectively employed bovine pericardium, chemically treated dura mater prostheses, porcine small intestinal submucosa, or the umbilical cord reinforced with polypropylene mesh [47, 48].

Biocompatible extracellular matrices, either single or double layer, composed of type I collagen derived from the bovine Achilles tendon, were experimentally used to cover defects in the abdominal wall or to shield intestinal loops from the aggression of meconium (intrauterine) in cases of gastroschisis, both prenatally and postnatally [49]. On these molds, the host cells will proliferate, break down the mold, and create autologous tissue (skin or even the abdominal wall) to cover the defect. This will prevent the intestinal loops from being altered at birth and make repairing the wall defect much simpler. By surgically eviscerating the fetal loops and inserting a collagen matrix in utero, a study in lambs also demonstrates that the intestinal loops return to the peritoneal cavity under the pressure of the contracting matrix and the enlargement of the loops. This creates pressure on the peritoneal cavity, which progressively increases its volume, simulating postnatal treatment with a silo-bag. Furthermore, the matrix was filled with host cells, which resulted in the autologous tissue covering the loops, shielding them from the damaging effects of the amniotic fluid during the final trimester. Postnatally, it was easy to close the wall defect and reinsert the remaining eviscerated loops into the abdominal cavity [49].

It has been shown that continuous negative pressure suction therapy (vacuum-assisted closure—VAC) for AWDs promotes the growth of granulation tissue, reduces infection and fluid loss, and speeds up wound healing (**Figure 10**). By stretching the abdominal wall and reducing the edema of the herniated viscera, negative pressure therapy also facilitates the viscera's return to the abdominal cavity [50, 51]. In newborns with large omphalocele and certain gastroschisis cases, VAC is a technically feasible and promising addition to the stepwise gravity reduction approach [50, 52].

Because the postoperative results are similar, the surgical solution for gastroschisis will only consider the degree of viscero-abdominal disproportion and the association of intestinal anomalies. However, to prevent abdominal compartment syndrome, intra- and postoperative intra-abdominal pressure monitoring will be required.

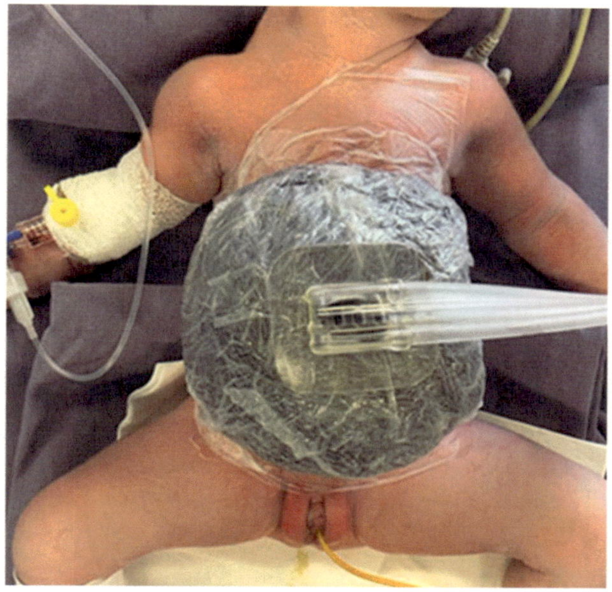

Figure 10.
VAC method for congenital AWDs.

12. Postoperative care

Patients need intensive therapeutic support in the immediate postoperative period, which includes nasogastric drainage and complete parenteral nutrition. Following each surgical procedure, arterial oxygen saturation, hydro-electrolyte balance, metabolic acidosis, base deficiency, lactatemia, and glycemia will be routinely assessed. Intubation and mechanical ventilation are typically maintained for 1–12 days after surgery, until all prosthetic materials are removed, the fascia is closed, or the abdominal defect is covered with skin. In certain cases, patients may need to return to the operating room right away if they exhibit symptoms of respiratory acidosis or a sudden change in hemodynamic status. If there is concomitant pulmonary hypoplasia, heart malformations, or preterm births, prolonged mechanical ventilation can also be required [53]. Since the lower limbs will probably be edematous and the blood at this level will be more concentrated in CO_2 and poorer in O_2, blood samples will ideally be taken from the upper limbs to monitor respiratory function.

The need to increase ventilatory pressures due to decreased diaphragm compliance, decreased venous return, cardiac output, ureteral obstruction, and oliguria can all be postoperative manifestations of abdominal compartment syndrome. For this reason, it is critical to monitor and maintain diuresis at 1 ml/kg/h, as well as central venous pressure, oxygen saturation, and perform chest X-rays [54].

Intravenous antibiotics will only be given during the initial days following primary closure of the anterior AWD, or if another surgical treatment option is being used, until the wall has completely closed. Every day, the surgical site is cleaned, covered with antibiotic ointment, and the sutures are removed 3 weeks later. Because the risk of wound infection and sepsis increases with the presence of an ileostomy in cases of concomitant intestinal atresia, proper management of the ileostomy and the use of leak-proof collection devices are essential. In most cases, the newborn will benefit from sedative-analgesia combining morphine with short doses of benzodiazepines based on needs; long-term curarization is rarely necessary.

The daily caloric intake *via* parenteral nutrition using a central venous catheter will be between 110 and 130 kcal/kg. Enteral nutrition will be gradually initiated after the nasogastric drainage is quantitatively reduced, no longer bilious, intestinal transit is resumed, intestinal loops are correctly aerated on the plain abdominal radiograph, and intestinal motility returns to normal: in a few weeks (usually 2–3 weeks) or even months for complex gastroschisis.

The sucking and swallowing reflexes, which may weaken while awaiting the return of intestinal transit, should be maintained by early oral stimulation. Additionally, intestinal pseudo-obstruction is occasionally linked to gastroschisis, which makes the restart of intestinal transit much more challenging [55]. Compared to children with simple gastroschisis, children with complex gastroschisis have a far higher risk of intestinal failure and bowel obstruction. The majority of the incidents took place in the first 2 years of life. Contrast examinations of the upper and lower digestive tract will be used to check for any potential intestinal atresia that was not initially noticed, if the patient is unable to tolerate meals and does not resume bowel movements after 3 weeks.

About 20% of patients with gastroschisis develop necrotizing enterocolitis, a common consequence that is strongly linked to the length of time they receive parenteral nutrition. Breast milk and natural feeding can lower this risk and significantly reduce the time to discharge from initiation of enteral nutrition [56].

13. Postoperative complications and long-term prognosis

Prematurity, abnormalities of the gastrointestinal tract, primary tension closure of the abdominal wall, and surgical site infections may all have a strong influence on postoperative complications [41]. Preventing issues with prematurity, hypothermia, respiratory distress, hyperbilirubinemia, hypoglycemia, and hypocalcemia is crucial because of the increased need for fluid intake and the delayed recovery of intestinal function in these children. Complications in treating anterior AWDs are less common as the medical-surgical team gains expertise and the neonatal critical care unit is more organized.

Although they cannot be directly linked to the patient's initial condition or the therapeutic approach used, infectious complications are the cause of these patients' elevated morbidity and death [57]. Intestinal peristalsis is reduced for a variable amount of time following abdominal wall surgery, ranging from a few days to a few weeks, and there is a risk of liver damage due to long-term parenteral nutrition. Although they are more common in individuals with gastroschisis in the first year of life, intestinal occlusions caused by adhesions or volvulus can theoretically occur at any age. According to different experts, between 6 and 20% of patients with anterior abdominal wall abnormalities undergo surgical reoperations for intestinal occlusions [58].

A relatively uncommon but very dangerous adverse consequence of gastroschisis linked to intestinal atresia, volvulus, or severe intestinal necrosis in the setting of necrotizing enterocolitis is short bowel syndrome. Long-term parenteral nutrition is necessary for short bowel syndrome, which is linked to infection risks, metabolic abnormalities, liver damage, and eventually the necessity for intestinal transplantation.

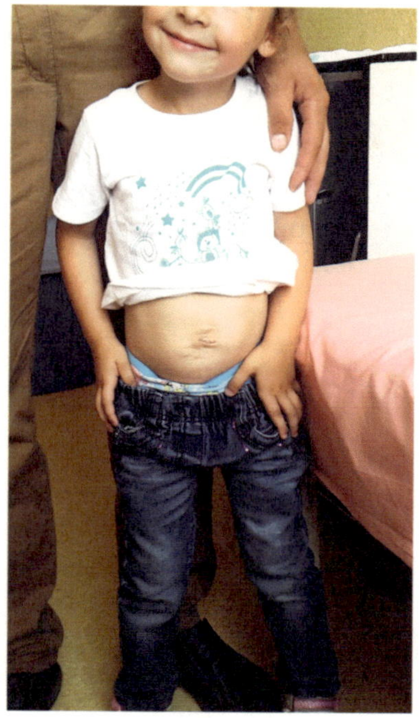

Figure 11.
Normal physical and intellectual development of a gastroschisis patient (7 years of age).

In the 1960s, the mortality rate for congenital anterior abdominal wall abnormalities was 90%; however, after 1990, it dropped to 2–10% and then to 5% for gastroschisis after 2000 [58, 59]. Complex gastroschisis, which is linked to intestinal atresia, volvulus, loop perforation or necrosis, intra-abdominal infections and sepsis, digestive hemorrhage, abdominal compartment syndrome, and respiratory distress, has a greater morbidity and death rate.

In around 90% of cases, children with gastroschisis have a very favorable long-term prognosis, which is dependent on the intestinal state at birth and whether intestinal atresia is present or not. Physical and intellectual development may be somewhat delayed in the first few years of life, but this decreases with age (**Figure 11**). Adult patients with congenital abdominal wall abnormalities have a normal quality of life and are socially and educationally adapted, according to standard questionnaires [60].

To avoid any unfavorable cosmetic appearance, whenever possible, an umbilicoplasty will be performed along with the primary closure of the AWD. Because physical appearance is a very important aspect today, especially in adolescents, excision of unsightly scars and umbilicoplasty will be scheduled as surgical interventions after the age of 5. For creating a natural-looking umbilicus, several surgical techniques may be used: C-V flap technique, umbilical stump reconstruction, a purse-string technique, or a modified "Y" or "Omega" flaps.

14. Conclusions

Although there is no consensus on certain aspects related to the optimal timing and mode of delivery, medical and surgical management as quickly as possible (within the first 6 hours of life), in a tertiary neonatal intensive care unit, can ensure a survival rate of over 90% in the case of gastroschisis. Surgical treatment, namely the integration of the intestinal loops into the abdomen and the closure of the anterior AWD, will be performed either per primam or in stages, depending on the complexity of the case and the degree of viscero-abdominal disproportion. Approximately 90% of children with anterior AWDs will benefit from normal physical, mental, and intellectual development and be able to fully integrate into society as adults if they do not have any associated abnormalities or deformities.

Conflict of interest

The author declares no conflict of interest.

Ethical approval

All photos are from the author's archive, taken from patients hospitalized and treated in the Pediatric Surgery Clinic of the "Sfânta Maria" Children's Emergency Hospital in Iasi, Romania; the photos were taken with the informed consent of the parents, and with the approval of the Ethics Committee of the "Sfânta Maria" Children's Emergency Hospital.

Author details

Elena Țarcă
Department of Surgery II, Discipline of Pediatric Surgery and Orthopedics, University of Medicine and Pharmacy "Gr.T.Popa", University Street, Iasi, Romania

*Address all correspondence to: tarca.elena@umfiasi.ro

References

[1] Bernstein P. Gastroschisis: A rare teratological condition in the newborn. Archives de Pédiatrie. 1940;**57**:505-513

[2] Reed EN. Infant disemboweled at birth: Appendectomy successful. JAMA. 1913;**61**:199

[3] Moore TC, Stokes GE. Report of two cases treated by a modification of the gross operation for omphalocele. Surgery. 1953;**33**:112-119

[4] Georgeades C, Mowrer A, Ortega G, Abdullah F, Salazar JH. Improved mortality of patients with gastroschisis: A historical literature review of advances in surgery and critical care from 1960-2020. Children (Basel). 2022;**9**(10):1504. Published 2022 Sep 30. DOI: 10.3390/children9101504

[5] Hoyme HE, Higginbottom MC, Jones KL. The vascular pathogenesis of gastroschisis: Intrauterine interruption of the omphalomesenteric artery. The Journal of Pediatrics. 1981;**98**:228-231

[6] Glick PL, Harrison MR, Adzick NS, Filly RA, de Lorimier AA, Callen PW. The missing link in the pathogenesis of gastroschisis. Journal of Pediatric Surgery. 1985;**20**(4):406-409. DOI: 10.1016/s0022-3468(85)80229-3

[7] Folkerth RD, Habbe DM, Boyd TK, McMillan K, Gromer J, Sens MA, et al. Gastroschisis, destructive brain lesions, and placental infarction in the second trimester suggest a vascular pathogenesis. Pediatric and Developmental Pathology. 2013;**16**(5):391-396

[8] Guanà R, Marocco L, Garofalo S, Zambaiti E, Pane A, Scottoni F, et al. A case of vanishing gastroschisis with short bowel syndrome treated by total parenteral nutrition and intestinal lengthening procedures. SAGE Open Medical Case Reports. 2023;**11**:2050313X231157490. DOI: 10.1177/2050313X231157490

[9] Palatnik A, Loichinger M, Wagner A, Peterson E. The association between gestational age at delivery, closure type, and perinatal outcomes in neonates with isolated gastroschisis. The Journal of Maternal-Fetal & Neonatal Medicine. 2020;**33**(8):1393-1399. DOI: 10.1080/14767058.2018.1519538

[10] Molik KA, Gingalewski CA, West KW, Rescorla FJ, Scherer LR, Engum SA, et al. Gastroschisis: A plea for risk categorization. Journal of Pediatric Surgery. 2001;**36**(1):51-55. DOI: 10.1053/jpsu.2001.20004

[11] Bielicki IN, Somme S, Frongia G, Holland-Cunz SG, Vuille-Dit-Bille RN. Abdominal wall defects-current treatments. Children (Basel). 2021;**8**(2):170. DOI: 10.3390/children8020170

[12] Raitio A, Lahtinen A, Syvänen J, Kemppainen T, Löyttyniemi E, Gissler M, et al. Gastroschisis in Finland 1993 to 2014-increasing prevalence, high rates of abortion, and survival: A population-based study. European Journal of Pediatric Surgery. 2020;**30**(6):536-540. DOI: 10.1055/s-0039-3401797. Epub 2019 Dec 31

[13] Țarcă E, Roșu ST, Cojocaru E, Trandafir L, Luca AC, Lupu VV, et al. Statistical analysis of the main risk factors of an unfavorable evolution in gastroschisis. Journal of Personalized Medicine. 2021;**11**(11):1168. DOI: 10.3390/jpm11111168

[14] Schuh JM, Cabacungan E, Wagner AJ. Birth prevalence of gastroschisis in the United States: 2016-2022. Pediatrics. 2025;**155**(4):e2024068696. DOI: 10.1542/peds.2024-068696

[15] Black AJ, Lu DY, Yefet LS, Baird R. Sex differences in surgically correctable congenital anomalies: A systematic review. Journal of Pediatric Surgery. 2020;**55**(5):811-820. DOI: 10.1016/j.jpedsurg.2020.01.016

[16] Baldacci S, Santoro M, Mezzasalma L, Pierini A, Coi A. Medication use during pregnancy and the risk of gastroschisis: A systematic review and meta-analysis of observational studies. Orphanet Journal of Rare Diseases. 2024;**19**(1):31. Published 2024 Jan 30. DOI: 10.1186/s13023-023-02992-z

[17] Materna-Kiryluk A, Więckowska B, Wiśniewska K, Czyżewska M, Godula-Stuglik U, Baumert M, et al. Geospatial clustering of gastroschisis in Poland: Data from the polish registry of congenital malformations (PRCM). International Journal of Occupational Medicine and Environmental Health. 2016;**29**(3):461-470

[18] Brender JD, Weyer PJ. Agricultural compounds in water and birth defects. Current Environmental Health Reports. 2016;**3**(2):144-152. DOI: 10.1007/s40572-016-0085-0

[19] Țarcă E, Roșu ST, Cojocaru E, Trandafir L, Luca AC, Rusu D, et al. Socio-epidemiological factors with negative impact on infant morbidity, mortality rates, and the occurrence of birth defects. Healthcare (Basel). 2021;**9**(4):384. DOI: 10.3390/healthcare9040384

[20] Muniz TD, Rolo LC, Araujo JE. Gastroschisis: Embriology, pathogenesis, risk factors, prognosis, and ultrasonographic markers for adverse neonatal outcomes. Journal of Ultrasound. 2024;**27**(2):241-250. DOI: 10.1007/s40477-024-00887-8

[21] Grossman M, Fischermann EA, German J. Sonographic findings in gastroschisis. Journal of Clinical Ultrasound. 1978;**6**(3):175-176

[22] Sezen P, Prayer F, Prayer D, Kasprian G, Metzelder M. Is fetal magnetic resonance imaging volumetry of eventrated organs in gastroschisis predictive for surgical treatment? Pediatric Radiology. 2021;**51**(10):1818-1825. DOI: 10.1007/s00247-021-05066-z

[23] Oakes MC, Porto M, Chung JH. Advances in prenatal and perinatal diagnosis and management of gastroschisis. Seminars in Pediatric Surgery. 2018;**27**(5):289-299. DOI: 10.1053/j.sempedsurg.2018.08.006

[24] Hakguder G, Olguner M, Gürel D, Akgür FM, Flake AW. Induction of fetal diuresis with intraamniotic furosemide injection reduces intestinal damage in a rat model of gastroschisis. European Journal of Pediatric Surgery. 2011;**21**(3):183-187. DOI: 10.1055/s-0031-1271708

[25] Callejas GH, Figueira RL, Gonçalves FLL, Volpe FAP, Zuardi AW, Crippa JA, et al. Maternal administration of cannabidiol promotes an anti-inflammatory effect on the intestinal wall in a gastroschisis rat model. Brazilian Journal of Medical and Biological Research. 2018;**51**(5):e7132. DOI: 10.1590/1414-431X20177132

[26] Feng C, Graham CD, Connors JP, Brazzo J 3rd, Pan AH, Hamilton JR, et al. Transamniotic stem cell therapy (TRASCET) mitigates bowel damage in a model of gastroschisis. Journal of

Pediatric Surgery. 2016;**51**(1):56-61. DOI: 10.1016/j.jpedsurg.2015.10.011. Epub 2015 Oct 22

[27] Kalache KD, Bierlich A, Hammer H, Bollmann R. Is unexplained third-trimester intrauterine death of fetuses with gastroschisis caused by umbilical cord compression due to acute extra-abdominal bowel dilatation? Prenatal Diagnosis. 2002;**22**(8):715-717. DOI: 10.1002/pd.386

[28] Landisch RM, Yin Z, Christensen M, Szabo A, Wagner AJ. Outcomes of gastroschisis early delivery: A systematic review and meta-analysis. Journal of Pediatric Surgery. 2017;**52**(12):1962-1971. DOI: 10.1016/j.jpedsurg.2017.08.068

[29] Kirollos DW, Abdel-Latif ME. Mode of delivery and outcomes of infants with gastroschisis: A meta-analysis of observational studies. Archives of Disease in Childhood. Fetal and Neonatal Edition. 2018;**103**(4):F355-F363. DOI: 10.1136/archdischild-2016-312394

[30] Blessed WB, Coughlin JP, Johnson MP, Evans MI, Jewell MR, Goyert GL, et al. Immediate delivery room repair of fetal abdominal wall defects. Fetal Diagnosis and Therapy. 1993;**8**(3):203-208. DOI: 10.1159/000263826

[31] Bianchi A, Dickson AP, Alizai NK. Elective delayed midgut reduction-no anesthesia for gastroschisis: Selection and conversion criteria. Journal of Pediatric Surgery. 2002;**37**(9): 1334-1336

[32] Sandler A, Lawrence J, Meehan J, Phearman L, Soper R. A "plastic" sutureless abdominal wall closure in gastroschisis. Journal of Pediatric Surgery. 2004;**39**(738):41. DOI: 10.1016/j.jpedsurg.2004.01.040

[33] Kronfli R, Bradnock TJ, Sabharwal A. Intestinal atresia in association with gastroschisis: A 26-year review. Pediatric Surgery International. 2010;**26**(9):891-894. DOI: 10.1007/s00383-010-2676-4

[34] Santos Schmidt AF, Goncalves A, Bustorff-Silva JM, Oliveira-Filho AG, Miranda ML, Oliveira ER, et al. Monitoring intravesical pressure during gastroschisis closure. Does it help to decide between delayed primary or staged closure? The Journal of Maternal-Fetal & Neonatal Medicine. 2012;**25**(8):1438-1441. DOI: 10.3109/14767058.2011.640366. Epub 2012 Apr 25

[35] Olesevich M, Alexander F, Khan M, Cotman K. Gastroschisis revisited: Role of intraoperative measurement of abdominal pressure. Journal of Pediatric Surgery. 2005;**40**:789-792

[36] Thompson RJ, Jaffray B. Gastric tonometry after gastroschisis repair. Archives of Disease in Childhood. 2002;**87**(4):339-340

[37] Schuster SR. A new method for the staged repair of large omphaloceles. Surgery, Gynecology & Obstetrics. 1967;**125**:837-850

[38] Allen RG, Wrenn EL. Silon as a sac in the treatment of omphalocele and gastroschisis. Journal of Pediatric Surgery. 1969;**4**:3-8

[39] Bhatnagar V, Das K, Agarwala S, Mitra DK. Silo construction from a sterile adhesive film and polypropylene mesh in the repair of gastroschisis and omphalocele. Pediatric Surgery International. 2001;**17**(5-6):356-358

[40] Burgos CM, Irvine W, Vivanti A, Conner P, Machtejeviene E, Peters N, et al. European reference network for rare inherited congenital anomalies

(ERNICA) evidence-based guideline on the management of gastroschisis. Orphanet Journal of Rare Diseases. 2024;**19**(1):60. DOI: 10.1186/s13023-024-03062-8

[41] Țarcă E, Cojocaru E, Trandafir LM, Melinte Popescu MG, Luca AC, Butnariu LI, et al. Nosocomial infections affecting newborns with abdominal wall defects. Healthcare (Basel). 2023;**11**(8):1131. DOI: 10.3390/healthcare11081131

[42] Henrich K, Huemmer HP, Reingruber B, Weber PG. Gastroschisis and omphalocele: Treatments and long-term outcomes. Pediatric Surgery International. 2008;**24**(2):167-173. DOI: 10.1007/s00383-007-2055-y

[43] Schlatter M, Norris K, Uitvlugt N, DeCou J, Connors R. Improved outcomes in the treatment of gastroschisis using a preformed silo and delayed repair approach. Journal of Pediatric Surgery. 2003;**38**(3):459-464. DOI: 10.1053/jpsu.2003.50079

[44] Charlesworth P, Akinnola I, Hammerton C, Praveena P, Desai A, Patel S, et al. Preformed silos versus traditional abdominal wall closure in gastroschisis: 163 infants at a single institution. European Journal of Pediatric Surgery. 2014;**24**(1):88-93. DOI: 10.1055/s-0033-1357755. Epub 2013 Oct 25

[45] Hawkins RB, Raymond SL, St. Peter SD, Downard CD, Qureshi FG, Renaud E, et al. Immediate versus silo closure for gastroschisis: Results of a large multicenter study. Journal of Pediatric Surgery. 2020;**55**(7):1280-1285. DOI: 10.1016/j.jpedsurg.2019.08.002. Epub 2019 Aug 22

[46] Gross RE. A new method for surgical treatment of large omphaloceles. Surgery. 1948;**24**:277-292

[47] Gabriel A, Gollin G. Management of complicated gastroschisis with porcine small intestinal submucosa and negative pressure wound therapy. Journal of Pediatric Surgery. 2006;**41**(11):1836-1840. DOI: 10.1016/j.jpedsurg.2006.06.050

[48] van Tuil C, Saxena AK, Willital GH. Experience with the management of anterior abdominal wall defects using bovine pericard. Hernia. 2006;**10**(1):41-47. DOI: 10.1007/s10029-005-0037-3

[49] Roelofs LA, Geutjes PJ, Hulsbergen-van de Kaa CA, Eggink AJ, van Kuppevelt TH, Daamen WF, et al. Prenatal coverage of experimental gastroschisis with a collagen scaffold to protect the bowel. Journal of Pediatric Surgery. 2013;**48**(3):516-524. DOI: 10.1016/j.jpedsurg.2012.07.056

[50] Butler MW, Fuchs J, Bruzoni M. Serial reduction of an extremely large gastroschisis using vacuum-assisted closure. European Journal of Pediatric Surgery Reports. 2018;**6**(1):e97-e99. DOI: 10.1055/s-0038-1676045

[51] Thanh Tri T, Minh Duc N, Phi Duy H, Thanh Thien N, Nguyen An Thuan L, Bang TL, et al. A case series describing vacuum-assisted closure for complex congenital abdominal wall defects. La Clinica Terapeutica. 2021;**172**(4):273-277. DOI: 10.7417/CT.2021.2331

[52] Nissen M, Romanova A, Weigl E, Petrikowski L, Alrefai M, Hubertus J. Vacuum-assisted staged omphalocele reduction: A preliminary report. Frontiers in Pediatrics. 2022;**10**:1053568. Published 2022 Nov 24. DOI: 10.3389/fped.2022.1053568

[53] Puvabanditsin S, Burger R, Puthenpura V, Walzer L, Madubuko A, Minerowicz C, et al. A giant gastroschisis

associated with pulmonary hypoplasia and spinal anomaly: A case report and a literature review. Case Reports in Pathology. 2018;**2018**:8378769. DOI: 10.1155/2018/8378769

[54] Baerg J, McAteer J, Miniati D, Somme S, Slidell M, American Pediatric Surgical Association Outcomes and Evidence-based Practice Committee. Improving outcomes for uncomplicated gastroschisis: Clinical practice guidelines from the American Pediatric Surgical Association outcomes and evidence-based practice committee. Pediatric Surgery International. 2024;**40**(1):246. Published 2024 Aug 30. DOI: 10.1007/s00383-024-05819-5

[55] Caldeman C, Fogelström A, Wester T, Mesas Burgos C, Löf Granström A. Long-term gastrointestinal morbidity in patients born with gastroschisis: A national register-based cohort study. Journal of Pediatric Gastroenterology and Nutrition. 2024;**79**(5):983-990. DOI: 10.1002/jpn3.12366

[56] Gulack BC, Laughon MM, Clark RH, Burgess T, Robinson S, Muhammad A, et al. Enteral feeding with human milk decreases time to discharge in infants following gastroschisis repair. The Journal of Pediatrics. 2016;**170**:85-89. DOI: 10.1016/j.jpeds.2015.11.046. Epub 2015 Dec 15

[57] Del Bigio JZ, Tannuri ACA, Falcão MC, de Carvalho WB, Matsushita FY. Gastroschisis and late-onset neonatal sepsis in a tertiary referral center in Southeastern Brazil. Jornal de Pediatria. 2022;**98**(2):168-174. DOI: 10.1016/j.jped.2021.05.003. Epub 2021 Jun 18

[58] Risby K, Husby S, Qvist N, Jakobsen MS. High mortality among children with gastroschisis after the neonatal period: A long-term follow-up study. Journal of Pediatric Surgery. 2017;**52**(3):431-436. DOI: 10.1016/j.jpedsurg.2016.08.022

[59] Machaea SS, Chitnis MR, Nongena P. Prevalence of gastroschisis and its neonatal mortality in the Eastern Cape Province tertiary institutions. African Journal of Paediatric Surgery. 2023;**20**(1):46-50. DOI: 10.4103/ajps.ajps_178_21

[60] Kapapa M, Rieg T, Serra A. A comparative analysis of quality of life in children managed for omphalocele and gastroschisis. African Journal of Paediatric Surgery. 2024;**21**(3):178-183. DOI: 10.4103/ajps.ajps_140_22

Chapter 2

Comparative Management of Infantile Hypertrophic Pyloric Stenosis: Insights into Ramstedt's and Double 'Y' Pyloromyotomy

Aruna Kumar Dash, Pramod Kumar Mohanty and Ayush Kumar Dash

Abstract

Infantile hypertrophic pyloric stenosis (IHPS) is the most common cause of gastric outlet obstruction in infancy, in which the pyloric portion of the stomach becomes hypertrophied, leading to obstruction of gastric emptying. Vomiting frequently transpires quickly after eating and progressively becomes more frequent and severe as the condition advances. IHPS is a relatively common gastrointestinal disorder in infancy, with an estimated incidence of 1 to 2 per 1000 live births and a male predominance ranging from 2:1 to 5:1. Prompt diagnosis and timely surgical intervention are essential to prevent serious metabolic derangements such as hypo-chloremic and hypokalemic metabolic alkalosis. Pyloromyotomy, the definitive surgical treatment, remains the cornerstone of management and has an excellent prognosis when performed appropriately. The first successful surgery was performed by Dufour and Fredet, in which the hypertrophic pyloric muscle was longitudinally split and closed transversely. However, Ramstedt introduced extramucosal pyloromyotomy in 1912, which remains the gold standard for the surgical management of IHPS. Later, in 2009, Alalayet et al. introduced a new technique known as Alalayet's Double-Y pyloromyotomy, which they claimed to have a better functional outcome compared to Ramstedt's pyloromyotomy while maintaining a similar safety profile. Our study demonstrated that the Double-Y pyloromyotomy procedure provides a better functional outcome regarding vomiting and weight gain in the early postoperative period. This seems to be due to the wider opening of the pyloric canal at both ends. This chapter explores the pathophysiology, clinical features, and a comparative analysis of surgical approaches for IHPS.

Keywords: infantile hypertrophic pyloric stenosis (IHPS), Ramstedt's pyloromyotomy, Double 'Y' pyloromyotomypyloric, muscle hypertrophy, mucosal perforation, surgical modification, laparoscopic pyloromyotomy, minimally invasive pediatric surgery

1. Introduction

Pyloric stenosis, formally known as infantile hypertrophic pyloric stenosis (IHPS), is a disorder characterized by the abnormal narrowing of the tube between the stomach and the duodenum (the pylorus) due to hypertrophy of the pyloric muscle. The thickness results from hypertrophy and hyperplasia of the pyloric muscle, predominantly affecting the circular layers, while hypertrophy of the underlying mucosa causes a gradual obstruction of the gastric outlet, hindering the normal flow of stomach contents into the duodenum. Affected newborns generally exhibit projectile vomiting, a vigorous ejection of stomach contents devoid of bile. The non-bilious characteristic of vomiting results from a blockage located proximal to the duodenal entry of bile. Vomiting frequently transpires quickly after eating and may initially present infrequently, but progressively gets more frequent and severe as the condition advances [1]. **Figure 1** depicts the anatomical characteristics and clinical manifestations.

Infantile hypertrophic pyloric stenosis (IHPS) is a relatively common gastrointestinal disorder in infancy, with an estimated incidence of 1 to 2 per 1000 live births. The condition demonstrates a clear male predominance, affecting males approximately four times more frequently than females, with a range of 2:1 to 5:1. This gender disparity is not yet fully understood but is consistent across various populations and geographic regions. IHPS is primarily a disorder of infancy, with onset typically between 2 and 12 weeks of age, and is extremely rare in adults, where it may be associated with chronic peptic disease or other secondary causes rather than the primary hypertrophic form seen in infants [2, 3].

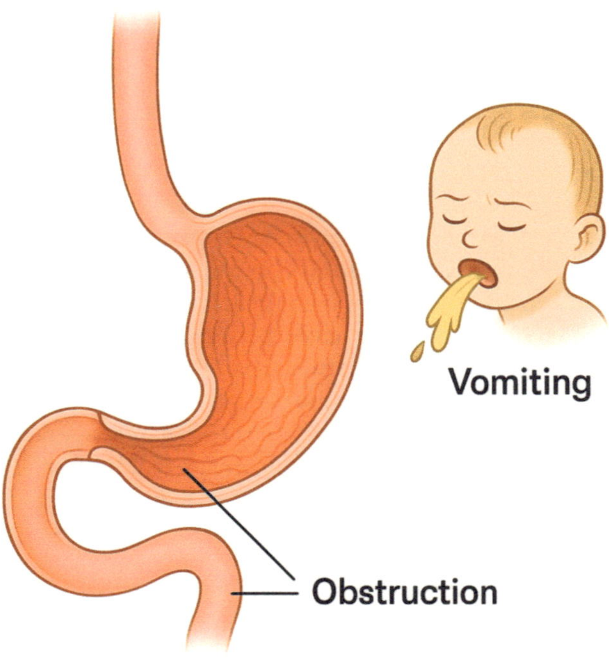

Figure 1.
Anatomical illustration of infantile hypertrophic pyloric stenosis (IHPS) showing thickened pyloric muscle leading to a narrowed pylorus, which obstructs gastric emptying and results in non-bilious projectile vomiting. This condition typically presents in early infancy and requires prompt medical evaluation and surgical correction.

Clinically, IHPS most frequently presents between the second and eighth week of life and is characterized by non-bilious projectile vomiting shortly after feeding. Affected infants may exhibit signs of dehydration, weight loss, and visible peristaltic waves across the abdomen. A palpable, firm, and mobile mass—commonly referred to as an "olive"—can often be felt in the right upper quadrant of the abdomen [4, 5].

Prompt diagnosis and timely surgical intervention are essential to prevent serious metabolic derangements such as hypochloremic, hypokalemic metabolic alkalosis [4, 5]. Pyloromyotomy, the definitive surgical treatment, remains the cornerstone of management and has an excellent prognosis when performed appropriately. This chapter explores pathophysiology, clinical features, and comparative surgical approaches for IHPS, with a focus on the classical Ramstedt's pyloromyotomy and the modified Double 'Y' pyloromyotomy techniques.

2. Etiology and contributing mechanisms

While most of the infantile hypertrophic pyloric stenosis (IHPS) cases occur sporadically, increasing evidence indicates a multifaceted etiology, characterized by a complex interaction of genetic predisposition, molecular dysregulation, and environmental factors. Familial clustering and sporadic instances of autosomal dominant inheritance indicate a heritable aspect; whereby certain infants may have genetic predispositions that are revealed by external factors such as early exposure to macrolide antibiotics or feeding practices that promote pyloric muscle hypertrophy [6–8].

IHPS may also present in syndromic disorders, often associated with congenital abnormalities impacting multiple organ systems. These relationships frequently arise from disturbances in the embryonic development of smooth muscle, neural innervation, or connective tissue structure, resulting in compromised peristalsis and heightened structural vulnerability in the pyloric area. At the molecular level, disruptions in intracellular signaling pathways—such as calcium flux regulation, cyclic nucleotide cascades, and mitogen-activated protein kinases (MAPKs)—have been associated with abnormal muscle cell proliferation and differentiation, leading to pathological thickening of the pyloric musculature. Furthermore, deficiencies in gap junction connection and receptor-ligand communication may hinder coordinated pyloric relaxation, worsening gastric outlet obstruction [9].

Recent data has underscored the significance of ciliopathies, wherein structural and functional abnormalities in primary cilia disrupt tissue morphogenesis and organ patterning, including that of the gastrointestinal tract. Similarly, irregularities in DNA repair processes, chromatin remodeling, and transcriptional regulation may disrupt cellular growth control at crucial stages of embryonic development, hence exacerbating aberrant pyloric muscle production [10].

Additionally, vascular and lymphatic abnormalities in the pyloric area can cause tissue congestion, hypoxia, and interstitial edema, leading to fibrotic remodeling and subsequent smooth muscle hypertrophy. These structural modifications, while not originating as primary factors, may synergistically interact with underlying genetic and molecular predispositions, hence increasing the likelihood of clinical disease. Prenatal environmental exposures, like maternal smoking, nutritional inadequacies, or teratogenic medication consumption, may act as precipitating factors that initiate the phenotypic expression of IHPS in genetically susceptible people [11–13].

Figure 2 demonstrates that the pathogenesis of IHPS is optimally understood as a multifaceted continuum, incorporating genetic, structural, molecular, and

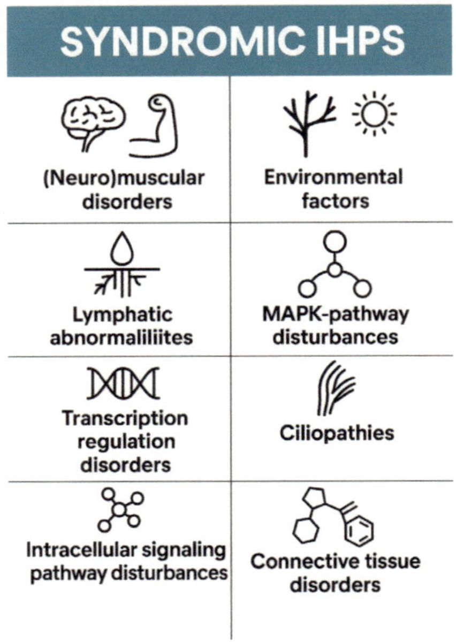

Figure 2.
Etiological factors associated with syndromic infantile hypertrophic pyloric stenosis (IHPS).

environmental factors. This intricacy emphasizes the need for a multidisciplinary diagnostic approach, especially in infants exhibiting the syndromic characteristics, and reinforces the significance of genetic counseling and coordinated care in these situations.

3. Pathological features of infantile hypertrophic pyloric stenosis

A critical biochemical outcome of chronic vomiting in IHPS is the onset of a distinctive hypochloremic, hypokalemic metabolic alkalosis. Recurrent vomiting results in significant loss of hydrochloric acid, depleting hydrogen and chloride ions from the bloodstream. This disturbance increases blood pH and reduces serum chloride, an essential ion necessary for bicarbonate excretion in the renal tubules. Without sufficient chloride, the kidneys cannot excrete excess bicarbonate, leading to increased alkalinity of the blood. Concurrently, fluid loss-induced volume depletion stimulates the renin-angiotensin-aldosterone system (RAAS), resulting in secondary hyperaldosteronism. This hormonal cascade facilitates sodium retention while enhancing the urine output of potassium and hydrogen ions, resulting in paradoxical aciduria, which exacerbates the pre-existing hypokalemia and metabolic alkalosis. As the alkalotic condition escalates, the body activates compensatory respiratory processes to reestablish acid-base equilibrium. Hypoventilation decreases minute ventilation, causing the respiratory system to hold carbon dioxide (CO_2), which reacts with water to produce carbonic acid (H_2CO_3), thus partially rectifying the increased blood pH. This compensation is biologically constrained, especially in neonates and babies, whose respiratory responses may be diminished or insufficient due to developmental immaturity. Therefore, it is essential to rectify the underlying fluid and electrolyte imbalances before proceeding with surgical intervention [14–16].

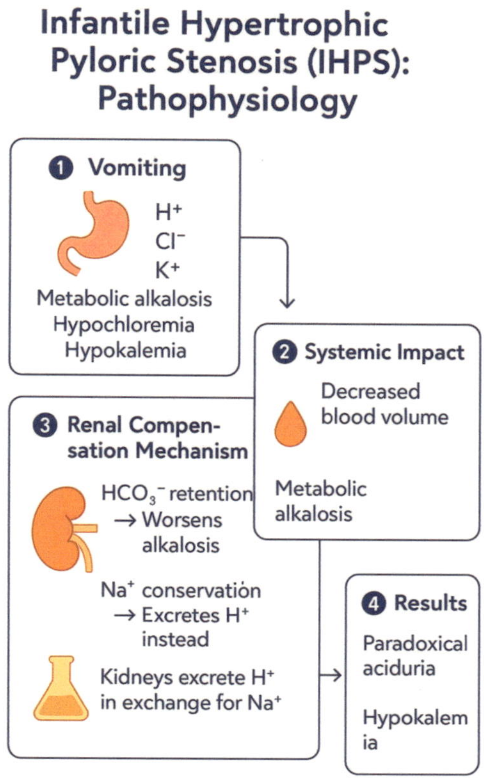

Figure 3.
Pathophysiological cascade of infantile hypertrophic pyloric stenosis (IHPS).

The pathophysiological cascade of IHPS includes mechanical obstruction and gastric dysmotility, as well as intricate systemic disturbances that extend beyond the gastrointestinal tract. The illness poses a complex clinical challenge due to cellular electrolyte alterations, endocrine activity, and respiratory compensation. Effective management necessitates timely identification and thorough stabilization to reduce the perioperative hazards. **Figure 3** illustrates the complex sequence of events, detailing the transition from pyloric muscle hypertrophy to metabolic and systemic disturbances, while highlighting the interrelation of gastrointestinal, renal, and respiratory physiology in the clinical progression of IHPS.

4. Diagnostic evaluation of infantile hypertrophic pyloric stenosis

The diagnosis of infantile hypertrophic pyloric stenosis (IHPS) necessitates a comprehensive, multimodal strategy that incorporates clinical evaluation, physical examination, diagnostic imaging, and laboratory analysis. Clinically, IHPS often manifests in newborns aged 3 to 12 weeks, characterized by non-bilious projectile vomiting, observable peristaltic waves in the left upper abdomen, and hypochloremic, hypokalemic metabolic alkalosis as the hallmark symptoms of IHPS: continued appetite despite emesis, inadequate weight gain, indications of dehydration, and heightened irritability. Postprandial emesis accompanied by paradoxical hunger is particularly indicative and acts as a crucial marker for early clinical suspicion [6].

During physical examination, a notable finding is the palpable "pyloric olive"—a hard, non-tender, movable mass generally situated in the epigastrium or right upper quadrant. This sign is optimally observed when the infant is tranquil and in a reclining position, typically after feeding, which alleviates abdominal tension. Moreover, apparent gastric peristalsis, albeit infrequently detected, may present as rhythmic waves moving from left to right across the epigastrium, indicative of the stomach's attempt to surmount the pyloric obstruction [17, 18].

Ultrasonography is esteemed as the primary imaging technique owing to its non-invasive characteristics, elevated sensitivity and specificity, and real-time anatomical representation. Definitive ultrasonographic requirements encompass a pyloric muscle thickness ranging from 3.5 mm (in premature newborns) to 4 mm or larger, alongside a channel length of 16 mm or more. Real-time imaging may further demonstrate the inability of stomach contents to transit into the duodenum. In ambiguous cases, or when sonographic results are indeterminate, an upper gastrointestinal (GI) contrast scan may be utilized, revealing characteristic features such as the "string sign" or "double track sign," both of which signify extension and constriction of the pyloric canal (**Figure 4**). Furthermore, sonographic evaluation of the spatial relationship between the superior mesenteric artery (SMA) and vein (SMV) is essential for ruling out intestinal malrotation, a potentially life-threatening differential diagnosis [19–21].

Laboratory examinations offer corroborative evidence by detecting the metabolic repercussions of prolonged vomiting, including hypochloremia, hypokalemia, and metabolic alkalosis. The biochemical changes illustrated in **Table 1** are induced by the depletion of stomach hydrochloric acid, the activation of secondary hyperaldosteronism, and transcellular potassium shifts. These findings not only bolster clinical suspicion but also significantly aid in directing preoperative fluid and electrolyte correction, which are crucial for reducing anesthesia-related risks and guaranteeing optimal surgical results [6].

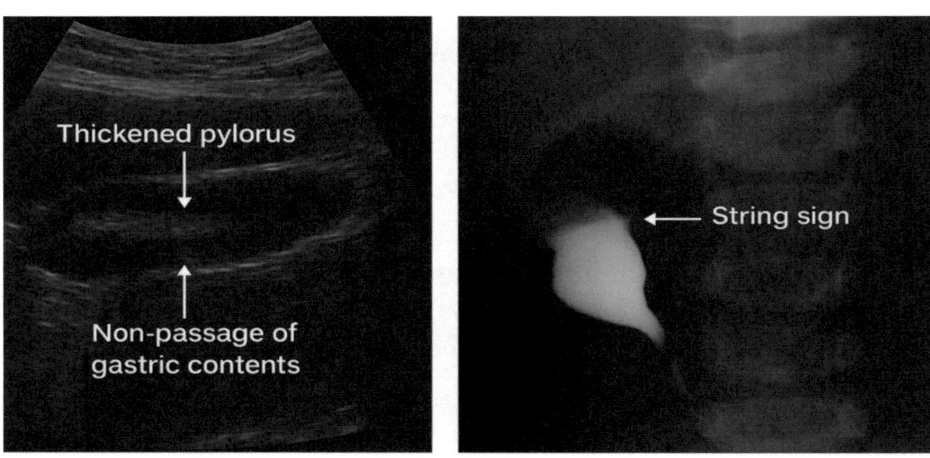

Figure 4.
Radiological findings in infantile hypertrophic pyloric stenosis (IHPS). Left: Ultrasonographic image showing a thickened pyloric muscle and non-passage of gastric contents, characteristic of IHPS. Right: Upper gastrointestinal contrast study (X-ray) demonstrating the classic "string sign," indicative of a narrowed and elongated pyloric channel due to muscular hypertrophy.

Parameter	Typical finding	Mechanism	Clinical implication
Serum chloride (Cl^-)	↓ Hypochloremia	Gastric HCl loss → impaired bicarbonate excretion	Promotes metabolic alkalosis
Serum potassium (K^+)	↓ Hypokalemia	Renal loss + intracellular shift via H^+/K^+ exchange	Risk of arrhythmia and neuromuscular dysfunction
Serum bicarbonate	↑ Elevated	Hydrogen ion loss + chloride depletion	Reflects metabolic alkalosis
Blood pH	↑ Alkalemia	Net gastric acid loss	Metabolic alkalosis
Arterial pCO_2	↑ Mildly Elevated	Hypoventilation (respiratory compensation for alkalosis)	Indicates partial respiratory compensation
Urine chloride	↓ Low	Renal conservation of chloride in hypochloremia	Marker of volume depletion and chloride loss

Table 1.
Common laboratory findings in IHPS.

5. Management of infantile hypertrophic pyloric stenosis

Although many non-surgical methods were tried, including frequent gastric lavage along with purgatives, the methods were largely unsuccessful. Use of atropine sulfate holds some promise to date but requires parenteral nutrition with prolonged hospital stay. It reduces muscle contraction and peristalsis, which in turn reduces spasm. The failure rate reported for atropine was 15–20% and the median hospital stay was 4–6 weeks. Most of the research concluded that atropine therapy should be restricted to only high-risk infants or in resource-poor settings where surgery on infants cannot be performed. It is worthwhile to mention that atropine is now being used as "rescue therapy" for incomplete surgical procedures where infants present with complaints after the initial procedure [22–24].

The conclusive treatment for infantile hypertrophic pyloric stenosis (IHPS) is surgical intervention. Pyloromyotomy is the usual curative treatment that alleviates blockage by incising the hypertrophied pyloric muscle. Ramstedt's pyloromyotomy has been a fundamental surgical procedure for decades, although recent innovations like the Double 'Y' pyloromyotomy have arisen to mitigate specific shortcomings of the conventional method. Both operations seek to restore stomach outflow, alleviate symptoms, and facilitate normal feeding and growth in afflicted newborns [6].

This flowchart outlines the primary surgical procedures used in the management of infantile hypertrophic pyloric stenosis (IHPS). Surgical intervention is the definitive treatment for IHPS, employing two primary techniques: Ramstedt's pyloromyotomy, the conventional and widely endorsed method that entails a longitudinal incision through the hypertrophied pyloric muscle; and the Double 'Y' pyloromyotomy, a modified approach aimed at enhancing muscle separation and minimizing the risk of mucosal damage. The selection of procedure is frequently influenced by the surgeon's proficiency, institutional guidelines, and particular intraoperative factors (**Figure 5**).

5.1 Traditional approach: Ramstedt's pyloromyotomy

Ramstedt's pyloromyotomy is the definitive procedure for the surgical treatment of infantile hypertrophic pyloric stenosis (IHPS). The operation, conducted using open (minimal laparotomy) or laparoscopic techniques, entails a longitudinal incision through the hypertrophied pyloric muscle to the submucosa, meticulously preserving the mucosa

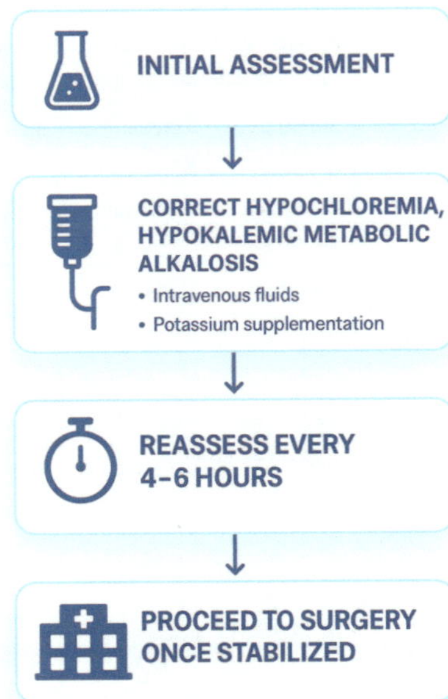

Figure 5.
Preoperative management algorithm for infantile hypertrophic pyloric stenosis (IHPS).

to alleviate gastric outlet obstruction. This procedure is preferred because to its technical simplicity, safety, and consistently positive results, as most infants can tolerate oral feeds within 6–12 hours postoperatively and are discharged within 48–72 hours [25].

Although medicinal treatments like atropine sulfate have demonstrated restricted efficacy in certain instances, surgery is the definitive global treatment, especially in achieving lasting symptom relief and normal feeding patterns [24].

A crucial factor in surgical success is preoperative physiological stabilization, especially the treatment of hypochloremic, hypokalemic metabolic alkalosis caused by prolonged vomiting. These metabolic changes provide considerable anesthetic risks, such as arrhythmias and hemodynamic instability, requiring extensive resuscitative interventions before surgery. Preoperative optimization entails the injection of N/2 saline (0.45% normal saline and 5% dextrose) to rectify volume depletion and sustain energy equilibrium and potassium chloride is added to mitigate hypokalemia. The restoration of serum chloride is crucial for bicarbonate elimination and the resolution of alkalosis. Stabilization generally transpires within 24–48 hours, necessitating vigilant monitoring of electrolytes, acid-base equilibrium, and hydration levels in babies. After stabilization, Ramstedt's pyloromyotomy is executed with minimal operational risk and a high probability of full recovery. Most newborns return to complete enteral eating within 1–2 days following surgery, with problems and recurrences being infrequent [26–29].

5.2 Modified technique: Double 'Y' pyloromyotomy

The Double 'Y' pyloromyotomy is an advanced surgical approach that modifies the traditional Ramstedt's surgery for addressing infantile hypertrophic pyloric stenosis (IHPS). This technique was developed to mitigate specific limitations of the conventional method, notably the risk of partial myotomy at the proximal and distal edges of the pyloric muscle and the possibility of mucosal damage resulting from restricted surgical exposure [30, 31].

In the Double 'Y' pyloromyotomy, two transverse incisions are incorporated—one at the proximal end and one at the distal end—of the conventional longitudinal pyloromyotomy. The incisions, in conjunction with the primary vertical cut, create a characteristic "Double Y" configuration. This arrangement considerably improves access to the full extent of the hypertrophied pyloric muscle, facilitating a more thorough and symmetrical division [31]. The enhanced visibility obtained using the Double 'Y' approach facilitates the identification of anatomical landmarks, diminishes the likelihood of residual obstruction, and lessens the danger of mucosal perforation. These benefits result in enhanced surgical precision, less intraoperative complications, and superior postoperative outcomes. Clinical observations indicate earlier tolerance of oral meals and reduced hospital stays in individuals using this modified method [32, 33].

The Double 'Y' pyloromyotomy approach, despite necessitating a somewhat steeper learning curve and a minor extension in operating duration, is increasingly acknowledged as a safe, successful, and technically superior alternative to the conventional procedure. It signifies the continuous advancement of pediatric surgical methodologies focused on improving results *via* increased procedural precision and patient safety [6].

5.3 Surgical procedure of Double 'Y' pyloromyotomy

The Double 'Y' pyloromyotomy is generally conducted under general anesthesia using either an open (minimal laparotomy) technique or a laparoscopic method, contingent upon the surgeon's preference and available institutional resources. The newborn is positioned supine with the right side slightly elevated to enhance access to the pyloric area. A transverse incision of approximately 2.5–3 cm in the right upper quadrant, positioned laterally to the lateral rectus, or a circum-umbilical approach, is employed to access the abdominal cavity [30, 31].

Upon identification and mobilization of the hypertrophied pylorus, it is carefully brought into the operating field. A longitudinal incision is performed on the anterior surface of the pyloric muscle, starting at the gastric antrum and extending to the proximal duodenum. The incision is meticulously deepened through the seromuscular layers until the underlying mucosa protrudes, indicating that the blockage has been alleviated without perforating the mucosa [34].

To attain the distinctive "Double Y" form, two supplementary transverse incisions are executed: one at the proximal end and another at the distal end of the longitudinal incision (**Figure 6**). These incisions enhance the surgical field and provide improved visibility of the complete muscle architecture. The muscle fibers are then delicately detached using a blunt instrument or pyloric spreader to finalize the myotomy. The mucosa must be distinctly observable along the whole length and width of the incision (**Figure 7**). The pylorus is relocated into the abdominal cavity, and the abdominal wall is sutured in layers with absorbable materials. Oral nutrition is often reinstated within 6 to 12 hours following surgery [35].

The above figures shows Double 'Y' pyloromyotomy, a modified surgical technique for the treatment of IHPS.

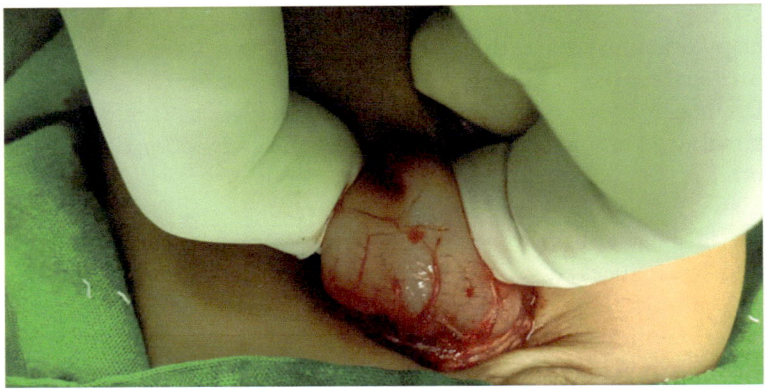

Figure 6.
Incision in case of Double Y pyloromyotomy.

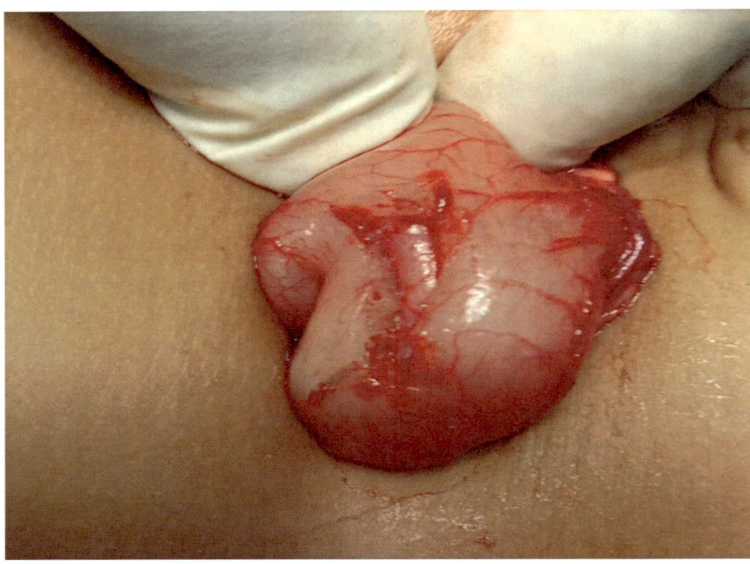

Figure 7.
After completion of Double-Y pyloromyotomy.

5.4 Advantages of the Double 'Y' technique

The Double 'Y' pyloromyotomy has numerous technical and therapeutic advantages over the traditional Ramstedt's technique. A key benefit is improved surgical visibility. The supplementary transverse incisions provide enhanced access to the pyloric muscle, especially at the frequently underexposed proximal and distal extremities. This enhanced visibility not only enables a more comprehensive and balanced muscle division but also diminishes the likelihood of residual obstruction—one of the primary problems associated with conventional pyloromyotomy. Furthermore, the approach markedly diminishes the probability of mucosal perforation. The enlarged field of view enables the surgeon to regulate dissection depth with more efficacy, thus enhancing surgical safety. Clinical observations suggest that patients who undergo the Double 'Y' procedure may experience a more rapid resumption of oral feeding and a reduced postoperative hospital duration, possibly attributable to fewer complications and more effective alleviation of blockage [35, 36].

5.5 Literature support and clinical evidence

An increasing body of data substantiates the therapeutic effectiveness of the Double 'Y' pyloromyotomy. Ordorica-Flores et al. [37] performed a prospective analysis revealing a reduced incidence of incomplete myotomy and improved postoperative results in patients utilizing the modified approach. Ohri et al. [38] observed a decrease in mucosal perforations, crediting this enhancement to the increased muscle exposure facilitated by the Double 'Y' shape. A systematic review and meta-analysis by Sola et al. [39] reported that the modified approach, including laparoscopic method, exhibited a more rapid resumption of complete oral feeding and a decreased duration of hospitalization. Oomen et al. [40] and Levy et al. [41] emphasized the need of surgical training in this method while underscoring its advantages in minimizing intraoperative errors and enhancing anatomical precision. Collectively, these studies highlight the Double 'Y' pyloromyotomy as a safe, effective, and potentially superior alternative to the traditional method, especially at facilities with pediatric surgical proficiency.

5.6 Comparative analysis of Ramstedt's and Double 'Y' pyloromyotomy techniques

Although Ramstedt's pyloromyotomy has historically been regarded as the gold standard in the surgical treatment of infantile hypertrophic pyloric stenosis (IHPS), advancements like the Double 'Y' pyloromyotomy have arisen as significant modifications intended to enhance surgical precision, exposure, and patient outcomes. The Double 'Y' approach enhances the traditional method by integrating transverse incisions at both the proximal and distal extremities of the longitudinal incision, creating a 'Y' shape. This modification improves vision and muscle accessibility, therefore overcoming the constraints associated with the old approach, such as partial myotomy and mucosal damage [42].

5.7 Surgical exposure and visualization

Ramstedt's approach utilizes a singular longitudinal incision above the hypertrophied pylorus, offering sufficient yet limited exposure. The Double 'Y' pyloromyotomy enhances access by extending the incision transversely at both the proximal and distal ends, so permitting thorough visibility of the pyloric borders. This increased exposure is especially advantageous for achieving thorough and uniform separation of the circular muscle fibers, particularly at anatomical extremities where residual hypertrophy may remain undetected [43].

This alteration enhances surgical vision and facilitates more controlled dissection, consequently diminishing intraoperative uncertainty and augmenting technical precision. The transverse extensions expand the operating field, facilitating improved manipulation of surgical instruments and minimizing the risk of excessive force that could jeopardize the underlying mucosa [44]. Moreover, enhanced anatomical clarity throughout the surgery may aid intraoperative decision-making, particularly in problematic situations such as borderline pyloric hypertrophy or anatomical variations. The enlarged field of vision facilitates precise evaluation of the myotomy's depth and breadth, guaranteeing that no portion of the pyloric ring is left unaddressed.

The statistically significant decrease in residual stenosis indicates that the Double 'Y' approach may serve a preventative function in postoperative problems, including prolonged vomiting, delayed stomach emptying, or the necessity for reoperation. Furthermore, improved visibility may decrease operating duration by obviating the necessity for frequent corrections or confirmations of myotomy thoroughness, thereby enhancing overall surgical efficiency [45].

5.8 Risk of incomplete myotomy and mucosal injury

The restricted visual and operating field associated with classic Ramstedt's pyloromyotomy may hinder visibility of the proximal and distal edges of the hypertrophied pyloric muscle, thereby elevating the risk of incomplete muscle division, especially at the anatomical extremes. This technical constraint leads to residual stenosis, a known cause of postoperative symptoms such recurrent vomiting or delayed stomach emptying, and, in rare instances, may require revision surgery [46].

The Double 'Y' pyloromyotomy resolves this issue by integrating transverse extensions at both extremities of the longitudinal incision, so enabling complete visibility of the circular muscle over its entire length. This structural modification facilitates accurate, full-thickness division under direct visualization, hence enhancing the uniformity and thoroughness of the myotomy. The expanded field diminishes the necessity for blind or forced dissection, hence mitigating the risk of unintentional mucosal breaches associated with the conventional method [47]. This enhanced anatomical access is associated with a quantifiable decrease in procedural difficulties. Recent observational studies and preliminary case series indicate a reduced rate of mucosal perforation, roughly 1.1% in Double 'Y' operations, compared to 4–5% in conventional Ramstedt's techniques. The disparity is both statistically significant and clinically relevant, considering the potential ramifications of mucosal injury, such as the necessity for surgical repair, extended hospitalization, and heightened risk of infection or leaking [27]. Moreover, the capacity to comprehensively visualize and regulate the degree of muscle division in the Double 'Y' technique may facilitate a reduced operating length, as it lessens the necessity for recurrent intraoperative evaluations or rectifications of incomplete incisions. From a system viewpoint, this results in enhanced surgical efficiency and less operating variability, particularly beneficial in high-volume pediatric facilities [6].

The advantages collectively highlight the Double 'Y' technique's potential to enhance patient safety, procedural effectiveness, and overall surgical outcomes, rendering it a persuasive alternative to the traditional procedure in suitable clinical contexts.

5.9 Precision and learning curve

Both Ramstedt's and Double 'Y' pyloromyotomy techniques yield favorable clinical outcomes when performed by proficient surgeons; however, the modified Double 'Y' method provides enhanced anatomical delineation, hence improving the precision and thoroughness of muscle dissection. The enhanced exposure and clarity of the pyloric borders enable more assured navigation of the surgical area, potentially reducing the possibility of residual hypertrophy or inadvertent mucosal damage [25]. Nonetheless, the benefits of this procedure must be weighed against its steeper learning curve, especially for surgeons familiar with the conventional single-incision method. The integration of bilateral transverse extensions necessitates a comprehensive comprehension of pyloric anatomy, alongside adeptness in the spatial alignment of muscle fibers and tactile feedback during dissection. Proficiency in this method necessitates intentional practice and is optimally facilitated by organized educational systems [12].

The inclusion of simulation-based training, encompassing high-fidelity cadaveric dissections, 3D-printed pyloric models, and virtual reality (VR)-assisted courses, can significantly enhance clinical acceptance. These modalities provide a risk-free setting for surgical trainees to cultivate essential motor skills, spatial awareness, and tissue-handling methods necessary for the safe performance of the Double 'Y' incision. Furthermore, this training can be incorporated into pediatric surgical fellowships and continuing medical education (CME) programs, guaranteeing proficiency and uniformity across institutions [48].

Three primary methods are utilized in the training of pediatric surgeons executing the Double 'Y' pyloromyotomy treatment for infantile hypertrophic pyloric stenosis (IHPS). Cadaveric dissection continues to be the benchmark for anatomical knowledge and hands-on education. 3D-printed anatomical models provide a consistent, economical resource for practical training, suitable for skill enhancement and spatial comprehension. Virtual reality (VR) platforms offer immersive, simulation-driven settings that facilitate repetitive procedural practice and cognitive mapping without danger to patients. These complimentary instruments collectively improve surgical expertise, diminish learning curves, and facilitate the safe implementation of advanced pyloromyotomy methods.

As minimally invasive surgical platforms advance, proficiency in anatomically intricate methods such as the Double 'Y' technique may improve adaptability to laparoscopic or robotic-assisted pyloromyotomy, where visual accuracy and meticulous dissection are essential. Consequently, investing in specialized training routes enhances surgical safety while also aligning with overarching objectives of innovation-driven, high-performance pediatric surgical care.

5.10 Postoperative recovery and complication rates

The Double 'Y' pyloromyotomy provides improved intraoperative visualization and more thorough muscle division, which is associated with a significantly reduced occurrence of postoperative problems such as persistent vomiting, delayed stomach emptying, and surgical site infections. The improved approach enhances the precision of myotomy, hence reducing the likelihood of residual pyloric blockage and mucosal injury, which are the significant factors in early postoperative morbidity [1, 2].

A significant clinical consequence linked to this method is the expedited resumption of enteral feeding. Research indicates that children who undergo Double 'Y' pyloromyotomy frequently accept oral feeds within 12 to 24 hours post-operatively, whereas those treated with the traditional Ramstedt's technique generally require 24 to 48 hours. This expedited meal schedule facilitates quicker gastrointestinal healing and diminishes the necessity for extended intravenous fluid administration or nasogastric decompression [27].

The abbreviated recovery trajectory correlates with a reduction in average hospital length of stay, which has wider implications for healthcare resource consumption. Premature discharge not only improves parental satisfaction—a vital indicator in pediatric surgical care—but also alleviates the strain on newborn intensive care units (NICUs) and related healthcare expenses. From a systems viewpoint, enhanced efficiency in postoperative management leads to increased patient throughput, reduced bed occupancy, and improved access for urgent or complex cases in crowded pediatric surgical centers [49]. Moreover, the decrease

Parameter	Ramstedt's pyloromyotomy	Double 'Y' pyloromyotomy
Surgical exposure	Linear incision; restricted field	Extended field *via* transverse incisions
Pyloric muscle visualization	Adequate; limited at extremes	Superior; full view of proximal and distal margins
Risk of incomplete myotomy	Higher at pyloric ends (2–5%)	Lower (<1%) due to expanded exposure
Mucosal perforation rate	4–5% (reported average)	1–2% (in modified techniques)
Postoperative vomiting	Occasional, resolves in 24–48 hrs	Lower incidence; faster resolution
Time to oral feeding	24–48 hours post-op	12–24 hours post-op
Hospital stay duration	2–3 days	Often reduced by 0.5–1 day
Learning curve	Well-established, familiar	Moderate; requires additional technique training
Suitability for MIS	Fully adaptable to laparoscopy	Under evaluation; promising but less standardized

Table 2.
Comparative summary table.

in complication rates and accelerated recovery may also lead to reduced readmission rates, improving both short- and long-term outcome profiles. These benefits advocate for the regular evaluation of the Double 'Y' modification, particularly in clinical settings where reducing hospital duration and enhancing surgical results are critically important (**Table 2**).

6. Clinical implications and future directions

In the advancing domain of minimally invasive pediatric surgery, innovations that enhance results without augmenting complexity are becoming increasingly significant. The Double 'Y' pyloromyotomy offers a technically advanced option that emphasizes exposure, accuracy, and minimized complication rates. Although widespread implementation necessitates systematic training and data from multicenter, randomized trials, preliminary clinical results indicate that the Double 'Y' approach may provide both immediate and enduring benefits, particularly in intricate or anatomically unclear situations.

Furthermore, its potential use in laparoscopic techniques and robot-assisted surgery necessitates additional research, especially in high-volume pediatric facilities aiming to reduce invasiveness while maintaining effectiveness.

7. Conclusion

Infantile hypertrophic pyloric stenosis is a medically treatable disorder with a high success rate. Although Ramstedt's pyloromyotomy remains prevalent, innovations like the Double 'Y' pyloromyotomy present possible enhancements in surgical results. Pediatric surgeons must stay abreast of advancing technology to customize procedures that optimally address individual patient requirements. This chapter emphasizes that the ultimate goal remains the same—effective relief of gastric outlet obstruction, rapid recovery, and minimal postoperative morbidity in infants afflicted with this condition.

Acknowledgements

Authors acknowledge the use of Grammarly for language polishing of the manuscript and Microsoft Copilot for reproducing animated figures and flow charts used as figures in the manuscript.

Author details

Aruna Kumar Dash[1*], Pramod Kumar Mohanty[1] and Ayush Kumar Dash[2]

1 Department of Pediatric Surgery, SVPPGIP, SCB Medical College, Cuttack, India

2 Department of Anatomy, Pabitra Pradhan Medical College, Talcher, India

*Address all correspondence to: dasharun02@gmail.com

References

[1] Ji Y, Lai X, Xu Z. Transumbilical single-site two incision laparoscopic pyloromyotomy for pediatric hypertrophic pyloric stenosis. BMC Surgery. 2022;**22**. DOI: 10.1186/S12893-022-01672-2

[2] Chalya PL, Manyama M, Kayange NM, Mabula JB, Massenga A. Infantile hypertrophic pyloric stenosis at a tertiary care hospital in Tanzania: A surgical experience with 102 patients over a 5-year period. BMC Research Notes. 2015;**8**:690. DOI: 10.1186/s13104-015-1660-4

[3] Krogh C, Gørtz S, Wohlfahrt J, Biggar RJ, Melbye M, Fischer TK. Pre- and perinatal risk factors for pyloric stenosis and their influence on the male predominance. American Journal of Epidemiology. 2012;**176**:24-31. DOI: 10.1093/aje/kwr493

[4] Abbas AE, Weiss SM, Alvear DT. Infantile hypertrophic pyloric stenosis: Delays in diagnosis and overutilization of imaging modalities. The American Surgeon. 1999;**65**:73-76

[5] Muse AI, Hussein BO, Adem BM, Osman MO, Abdulahi ZB, Ibrahim MA. Treatment outcome and associated factors of infantile hypertrophic pyloric stenosis at eastern Ethiopia public hospitals. BMC Surgery. 2024;**24**:262. DOI: 10.1186/S12893-024-02567-0

[6] Garfield K, Sergent SR. Pyloric Stenosis - StatPearls - NCBI Bookshelf. StatPearls, Treasure Island (FL): StatPearls Publishing; 2023

[7] Kumar R, Abel R. Infantile hypertrophic pyloric stenosis. Surgery (Oxford). 2005;**23**:323-325. DOI: 10.1383/SURG.2005.23.9.323

[8] Yang G, Brisseau G, Yanchar NL. Infantile hypertrophic pyloric stenosis: An association in twins? Paediatrics & Child Health. 2008;**13**:383. DOI: 10.1093/PCH/13.5.383

[9] Peeters B, Benninga MA, Hennekam RCM. Infantile hypertrophic pyloric stenosis--genetics and syndromes. Nature Reviews. Gastroenterology & Hepatology. 2012;**9**:646-660. DOI: 10.1038/NRGASTRO.2012.133

[10] Abdellatif M, Ghozy S, Kamel MG, Elawady SS, Ghorab MME, Attia AW, et al. Association between exposure to macrolides and the development of infantile hypertrophic pyloric stenosis: A systematic review and meta-analysis. European Journal of Pediatrics. 2019;**178**:301-314. DOI: 10.1007/S00431-018-3287-7

[11] Jedd MB, Melton LJ, Griffin MR, Kaufman B, Hoffman AD, Broughton D, et al. Factors associated with infantile hypertrophic pyloric stenosis. American Journal of Diseases of Children. 1988;**142**:334-337. DOI: 10.1001/ARCHPEDI.1988.02150030108033

[12] Obaid YY, Toubasi AA, Albustanji FH, Al-Qawasmeh AR. Perinatal risk factors for infantile hypertrophic pyloric stenosis: A systematic review and meta-analysis. Journal of Pediatric Surgery. 2023;**58**:458-466. DOI: 10.1016/J.JPEDSURG.2022.08.016

[13] Boybeyi-Turer O, Celik HT, Arslan UE, Soyer T, Tanyel FC, Kiran S. Environmental exposure in the etiology of infantile hypertrophic pyloric stenosis: A systematic review and meta-analysis. Pediatric Surgery International.

2022;**38**:951-961. DOI: 10.1007/s00383-022-05128-9

[14] Tutay GJ, Capraro G, Spirko B, Garb J, Smithline H. Electrolyte profile of pediatric patients with hypertrophic pyloric stenosis. Pediatric Emergency Care. 2013;**29**:465-468. DOI: 10.1097/PEC.0B013E31828A3006

[15] Dalton BGA, Gonzalez KW, Boda SR, Thomas PG, Sherman AK, Peter SD. Optimizing fluid resuscitation in hypertrophic pyloric stenosis. Journal of Pediatric Surgery. 2016;**51**:1279-1282. DOI: 10.1016/J.JPEDSURG.2016.01.013

[16] Panteli C. New insights into the pathogenesis of infantile pyloric stenosis. Pediatric Surgery International. 2009;**25**:1043-1052. DOI: 10.1007/S00383-009-2484-X

[17] Aspelund G, Langer JC. Current management of hypertrophic pyloric stenosis. Seminars in Pediatric Surgery. 2007;**16**:27-33. DOI: 10.1053/j.sempedsurg.2006.10.004

[18] Peters B, Oomen MWN, Bakx R, Benninga MA. Advances in infantile hypertrophic pyloric stenosis. Expert Review of Gastroenterology & Hepatology. 2014;**8**:533-541. DOI: 10.1586/17474124.2014.903799

[19] Park JS, Byun YH, Choi SJ, Lee JS, Ryu JM, Lee JY. Feasibility of point-of-care ultrasound for diagnosing hypertrophic pyloric stenosis in the emergency department. Pediatric Emergency Care. 2021;**37**:550-554. DOI: 10.1097/PEC.0000000000002532

[20] Olson AD, Hernandez R, Hirschl RB. The role of ultrasonography in the diagnosis of pyloric stenosis: A decision analysis. Journal of Pediatric Surgery. 1998;**33**:676-681. DOI: 10.1016/S0022-3468(98)90186-5

[21] van den Bunder FA, Derikx JP, Kiblawi R, van Rijn RR, Dingemann J. Diagnostic accuracy of palpation and ultrasonography for diagnosing infantile hypertrophic pyloric stenosis: A systematic review and meta-analysis. The British Journal of Radiology. 2022;**95**:20211251. DOI: 10.1259/bjr.20211251

[22] Lukac M, Antunovic S, Vujovic D, Pavicevic P, Jesic M, Krstajic T, et al. Is abandonment of nonoperative management of hypertrophic pyloric stenosis warranted? European Journal of Pediatric Surgery. 2013;**23**:80-84. DOI: 10.1055/S-0032-1333114

[23] Takeuchi M, Yasunaga H, Horiguchi H, Hashimoto H, Matsuda S. Pyloromyotomy versus i.v. atropine therapy for the treatment of infantile pyloric stenosis: Nationwide hospital discharge database analysis. Pediatrics International. 2013;**55**:488-491. DOI: 10.1111/PED.12100

[24] Yamataka A, Tsukada K, Yokoyama-Laws Y, Murata M, Lane GJ, Osawa M, et al. Pyloromyotomy versus atropine sulfate for infantile hypertrophic pyloric stenosis. Journal of Pediatric Surgery. 2000;**35**:338-342. DOI: 10.1016/S0022-3468(00)90036-8

[25] Ismail I, Elsherbini R, Elsaied A, Aly K, Sheir H, Laparoscopic vs. Open Pyloromyotomy in treatment of infantile hypertrophic pyloric stenosis. Frontiers in Pediatrics. 2020;**8**:426. DOI: 10.3389/FPED.2020.00426

[26] Campbell BT, McLean K, Barnhart DC, Drongowski RA, Hirschl RB. A comparison of laparoscopic and open pyloromyotomy at a teaching hospital. Journal of Pediatric Surgery. 2002;**37**:1068-1071. DOI: 10.1053/JPSU.2002.33846

[27] Kneen L. Pyloric stenosis. Pediatric Care. 2022. DOI: 10.1542/AAP.PPCQR.396220

[28] Ramji J, Joshi RS. Laparoscopic pyloromyotomy for congenital hypertrophic pyloric stenosis: Our experience with twenty cases. African Journal of Paediatric Surgery. 2021;**18**:14-17. DOI: 10.4103/AJPS.AJPS_119_20

[29] Shaw A. Ramstedt and the centennial of pyloromyotomy. Journal of Pediatric Surgery. 2012;**47**:1433-1435. DOI: 10.1016/j.jpedsurg.2012.06.002

[30] Alalayet YF, Miserez M, Mansoor K, Khan AM. Double-Y pyloromyotomy: A new technique for the surgical management of infantile hypertrophic pyloric stenosis. European Journal of Pediatric Surgery. 2009;**19**:17-20. DOI: 10.1055/S-2008-1039025

[31] Alalayet YF, Miserez M, Mansoor K, Khan AM. Double-Y pyloromyotomy: A new technique for the surgical management of infantile hypertrophic pyloric stenosis. European Journal of Pediatric Surgery. 2009;**19**:17-20

[32] Graham KA, Laituri CA, Markel TA, Ladd AP. A review of postoperative feeding regimens in infantile hypertrophic pyloric stenosis. Journal of Pediatric Surgery. 2013;**48**:2175-2179. DOI: 10.1016/j.jpedsurg.2013.04.023

[33] Georgeson KE, Corbin TJ, Griffen JW, Breaux CW. An analysis of feeding regimens after pyloromyotomy for hypertrophic pyloric stenosis. Journal of Pediatric Surgery. 1993;**28**:1478-1480. DOI: 10.1016/0022-3468(93)90435-n

[34] Parikh RM, Ata A, Edwards MJ. A contemporary review of surgical approach and outcomes in pediatric hypertrophic pyloric stenosis. The Journal of Surgical Research. 2023;**285**:142-149. DOI: 10.1016/J.JSS.2022.12.034

[35] Kelay A, Hall NJ. Perioperative complications of surgery for hypertrophic pyloric stenosis. European Journal of Pediatric Surgery. 2018;**28**:171-175. DOI: 10.1055/s-0038-1637016

[36] Dash AK, Sahoo R, Mohanty PK, Jena PK, Panda AK, Tripathy PK. To access the management and outcome of infantile hypertrophic pyloric stenosis by Ramstedt's Pyloromyotomy versus Double 'Y' Pyloromyotomy. African Journal of Paediatric Surgery. 2022;**20**:264. DOI: 10.4103/ajps.ajps_67_22

[37] Ordorica-Flores R, León-Villanueva V, Bracho-Blanchet E, Reyes-Retana R, Dávila-Perez R, Varela-Fascinetto G, et al. Infantile hypertrophic pyloric stenosis: A comparative study of pyloric traumamyoplasty and Fredet-Ramstedt pyloromyotomy. Journal of Pediatric Surgery. 2001;**36**:1000-1003. DOI: 10.1053/jpsu.2001.24724

[38] Ohri SK, Sackier JM, Singh P. Modified Ramstedt's pyloromyotomy for the treatment of infantile hypertrophic pyloric stenosis. Journal of the Royal College of Surgeons of Edinburgh. 1991;**36**:94-96

[39] Sola JE, Neville HL. Laparoscopic vs open pyloromyotomy: A systematic review and meta-analysis. Journal of Pediatric Surgery. 2009;**44**:1631-1637. DOI: 10.1016/j.jpedsurg.2009.04.001

[40] Oomen MWN, Hoekstra LT, Bakx R, Heij HA. Learning curves for pediatric laparoscopy: How many operations are enough? The Amsterdam experience with laparoscopic pyloromyotomy. Surgical Endoscopy. 2010;**24**:1829-1833. DOI: 10.1007/s00464-010-0880-x

[41] Levy BE, MacDonald M, Bontrager N, Castle JT, Draus JM, Worhunsky DJ. Evaluation of the learning curve for laparoscopic

pyloromyotomy. Surgical Endoscopy. 2023;**37**:5101-5108. DOI: 10.1007/s00464-023-09962-3

[42] Lunger F, Staerkle RF, Muff JL, Fink L, Holland-Cunz SG, Vuille-dit-Bille RN. Open versus Laparoscopic Pyloromyotomy for pyloric stenosis-a systematic review and meta-analysis. The Journal of Surgical Research. 2022;**274**:1-8. DOI: 10.1016/J.JSS.2021.12.042

[43] Pogorelić Z, Zelić A, Jukić M, Llorente Muñoz CM. The safety and effectiveness of Laparoscopic Pyloromyotomy using 3-mm electrocautery hook versus open surgery for treatment of hypertrophic pyloric stenosis in infants. Children (Basel). 2021:8. DOI: 10.3390/children8080701

[44] Zaghal A, El-Majzoub N, Jaafar R, Aoun B, Jradi N. Brief overview and updates on infantile hypertrophic pyloric stenosis: Focus on perioperative management. Pediatric Annals. 2021;**50**:e136-e141. DOI: 10.3928/19382359-20210215-01

[45] van den Bunder FAIM, Hall NJ, van Heurn LWE, Derikx JPM. A Delphi analysis to reach consensus on preoperative care in infants with hypertrophic pyloric stenosis. European Journal of Pediatric Surgery. 2020;**30**:497-504. DOI: 10.1055/s-0039-3401987

[46] Mazurak M, Patkowski D. A history of the surgical correction of pyloric stenosis. Journal of Pediatric Surgery. 2021;**56**:1904-1907. DOI: 10.1016/j.jpedsurg.2021.05.009

[47] Danielson J, Svenningsson A, Jansson P, Läckgren G. Controlled long term outcome of pyloromyotomy for pyloric stenosis: No long-term adverse effect. Journal of Pediatric Surgery. 2022;**57**:736-739. DOI: 10.1016/j.jpedsurg.2022.04.005

[48] Jiang Y, Jiang H, Yang Z, Li Y. The current application of 3D printing simulator in surgical training. Front Med (Lausanne). 2024;**11**:1443024. DOI: 10.3389/fmed.2024.1443024

[49] Staerkle RF, Lunger F, Fink L, Sasse T, Lacher M, von Elm E, et al. Open versus laparoscopic pyloromyotomy for pyloric stenosis. Cochrane Database of Systematic Reviews. 2021;**3**:CD012827. DOI: 10.1002/14651858.CD012827.pub2

Section 2

Pediatric Reconstructive Surgery

Chapter 3

Median Clefts of the Upper Lip

Luis Monasterio Aljaro, Alison Ford Martinez de Pinillos and Luis Fernando Monasterio Roman

Abstract

Our face serves as our personal presentation card to the world. It determines our appearance, how our peers see us, and reflects in the first instance the image we want to show to the world. Minor birth malformations occur in 71% of the head and neck. It is reasonable to think that most of these patients will experience changes in social adaptation to their environment. Although Median Cleft Lip (MCL) has a very low incidence, it accounts for 26.7% of atypical cleft lips.There is an incomplete fusion of the medial nasal prominences during the development of the embryo.The phenotypes shows a broad spectrum of clefts ranging from a simple vermillion notch to the more severe lesions in the lip and nose associated with intracranial malformations. DeMyer classification of MCL patients include two groups: 1. Hypoteleorbitisn (bad prognosis) and 2. Normo-Hiperteleoribitisn (good prognosis). The experience of 55 cases of the different types of MCL is shown, detailing classification, surgical management, prognosis, and long-term results. The understanding of its pathogenesis and development of the facial abnormalities is essential, to repair in time and avoid the psychosocial consequences for the individual.

Keywords: median cleft lip, holoprosencephaly, binderoid, abbe flap, hypoteleotbitism

1. Introduction

The aim of this Chapter is to show the experience in MCL of a senior plastic surgeon who devoted a long time to the treatment of patients with facial cleft and present an updated review of available information on the subject, including its pathophysiology, classifications, and management. Photographs illustrate different types of MCL and the results after the surgery.

2. Body of the manuscript

Congenital malformations are structural anomalies or defects observed at the moment of birth that may affect any place of the human body. The exact cause of MCL is unknown and may be associated with genetic and environmental factors, deficit of nutrients, use of drugs and alcohol, or viral diseases during the pregnancy. Cleft lips are a frequent malformation in humans; one in every 800–1000 newborn is usually unilateral or bilateral cleft lip. The MCL is uncommon, located in middle line of the upper lip, but it is not exclusive in humans; in some animals, you can observe median clefts of the upper lip, as a normal anatomical condition; the "hare lip "affects also camelids, felines, and marsupials.

"Any congenital and vertical cleft in the center of the upper lip, regardless of extension is an MCL" [1]. According to the Tessier classification [2], the MCL corresponds to a cleft in axis number 0. Atypical cleft lips are 1% of cleft lip population. The diverse types of Tessier facial clefts are presented in **Table 1**.

While its true incidence is not well determined, it is estimated that currently, MCL occurs in 1.4 to 4.9 per 100,000 live births. Authors and number of cases are in **Table 2**. Dr Ortiz Monasterio in his study of series of 345 patients with rare cleft,26.7% of them were MCL [3].

The study of 6500 cleft lips in Chile, attended for 30 years in Fundacion Gantz, 55 corresponded to MCL (0,8%). Recently, reference [4] has estimated an incidence between 0.43% and 0.73% of the total cleft population.

2.1 Pathogenesis

Regarding MCL, several theories have been proposed to explain the mechanism of the formation of a middle line cleft in the embryo. The two most classic theories correspond to the "Fusion Theory" proposed [5] in 1869, as a failure in the fusion of the facial process. The mesoderm and ectoderm union are done between the 3rd and 8 weeks. The complete formation of the upper lip is related to the fusion of the medial nasal prominence, lateral prominence, and medial aspect of the maxillary process. Another theory [6] that could explain the central cleft suggests failure in the cellular migration and penetration from the neural crest of the mesoderm in the middle line. The disruption in the nasofrontal process, of small units of growth, could account for

Tessier Cleft Number	Number of Clefts (%)
0	92 (26,7)
1	16 (4,7)
2	23 (6,7)
3	15 (4,4)
4	8 (2,3)
5	1 (0,3)
6	16 (4,6)
7	48 (13,9)
8	4 (1,2)
9	4 (1,2)
10	28 (8,1)
11	15 (4,4)
12	19 (5,5)
13	21 (6,1)
14	35 (10,2)

Table 1.
Distribution of atypical craniofacial clefts.

Year	Author	Country	Patients with cleft	Number of Median Cleft	Percentage (%)
1935	Davis	U.S.A.	688	5	0,7
1963	Knox	England	574	3	0,5
1965	Fogh-Andersen	Denmark	3940	15	0,4
1967	Tesserra	Spain	378	11	2,9
1974	Tessier	U.S.A.	336	14	4,1
1978	Irregbulem	Nigeria	70	3	4,2
1987	Ortiz-Monasterio	México	5586	92	1,6
2003	Mulliken	U.S.A.	695	6	1,1
2025	Monasterio	Chile	4680	55	0.8

Table 2.
Median Clefts Lip (MCL) casuistic over the years.

the midline cleft. Sulik [7] points to a variability in the location of the ossification centers; there is a disruption of small growth center units within the nasofrontal eminence.

Recently, Carstens [8] has proposed the "LEGO model" of craniofacial development, based on the existence of "development fields" that act as blocks to be merged to shape the final structure. A failure in one of these blocks (excess or deficiency) leads to failure in the assembly of the adjacent blocks. Each of these "development fields" consists of a neurovascular pedicle, with components of the neural crest, generating a specific subunit called Neuromere (development unit of early Central Nervous System).

According to Carstens, for the correct formation of craniofacial structures, certain requirements must be met. The first is that there must be a correct positioning and development of "growth cone" of each of the development fields, which should be at a critical distance contact. If for some reason the size and volume of the development fields is reduced and growth cones fail to develop as they should be, a greater distance between fields will exist, which will lead to the "no-fusion," and therefore, the cleft in the lip appears.

The second requirement involves proper activation of the epithelium of each field for merging correctly. The stability of the epithelium depends on a molecule called Sonic Hedgehog (SHH). While SHH is active, the epithelium will not merge. SHH is inhibited by BMP-4 (bone morphogenetic protein), which is produced by the mesenchyme in each field and is proportional to its volume. If BMP-4 is produced, SHH function is inhibited, allowing the epithelium fusion. Conversely, if the volume of a development field is small, it will produce less BMP-4, and therefore, SHH will be not inhibited, preventing epithelium fusion, thereby generating a cleft. More details of the complicated mechanisms involving the embryological development and anomalies are in the book published by Carstens [9] in 2023 "*Embryological basis of craniofacial structures developmental anatomy, evolutionary design and clinical applications*," a monumental and complete work, of 1.771 pages. Anyhow, the problem is in the middle area of growth or frontonasal process due to failure to complete the prolabial development.

A recent investigation [10] related to gene DISP1 has encoded a transmembrane protein that regulates the secretion of the morphogen, Sonic hedgehog, a deficiency of which is a major cause of HPC. The study was made in 25 individuals with midline craniofacial defects; a total of 23 DISP1 variants pathogenic were identified in these patients. The author's conclusion highlights the clinical risks to be flagged up during genetic counseling after the discovery of a pathogenic DISP1 variant.

2.2 Classification

There are several proposed classifications for MCL; standing out are DeMyer, Wu, and Mary de Boutry.

DeMyer [11, 12] classification sets two major groups in the MCL, depending on the distance between the orbits: I.-"hypoteleorbitism "(**Figure 1**) and group II.- "hyperteleorbitism- normoteleorbitism"(**Figure 2**).

The hypo group is associated with variable degrees of intracranial malformations; the most frequent and important is Holoprosencephaly (HPE).

HPE is the most common malformation of the prosencephalon in humans. It is characterized by a continuum of structural brain anomalies resulting from the failure of midline cleavage of the prosencephalon. The three classic subtypes of HPE are alobar, semilobar, and lobar, although a few additional categories have been added to this original classification. In cases of severe HPC, the premaxillary segments of the face remain unformed, causing midline facial defects, such as arrhinia, midline facial clefts, hypotelorism, and cyclopia The widely accepted classification system for HPE was proposed by DeMyer, who divided HPE into three subcategories: alobar, when there is a complete lack of separation of the cerebral hemispheres and a large mono-ventricle; semi-lobar, with only the anterior lobes failing to separate but the parieto-occipital regions divided by the interhemispheric fissure and falx cerebri; and lobar, when only the most rostral-inferior parts of the frontal lobes are fused. It is fundamental to keep in mind that HPC represents a continuum of forebrain malformations and no clear distinctions among these different categories should be expected. In cases of severe HPE, the premaxillary segments of the face remain unformed, causing midline facial defects. Initially divided into 5 groups: I. Cyclope, II. Otocephaly III., Cynocephaly, IV.MCL Hypotelerbitism with flat nose and midline cleft, absence of the premaxilla (**Figure 3**), group V. Hypotelerbitism flat nose and bilateral cleft lip. In **Table 3** is a summary of the diverse types of HPE.

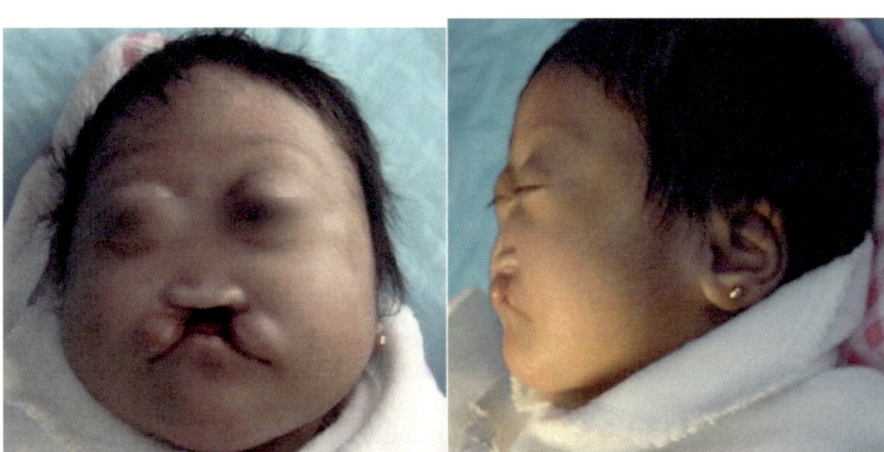

Figure 1.
Patient with hypotelorbitism MCL. Observe the short distance between the eyes and the extreme flat nose.

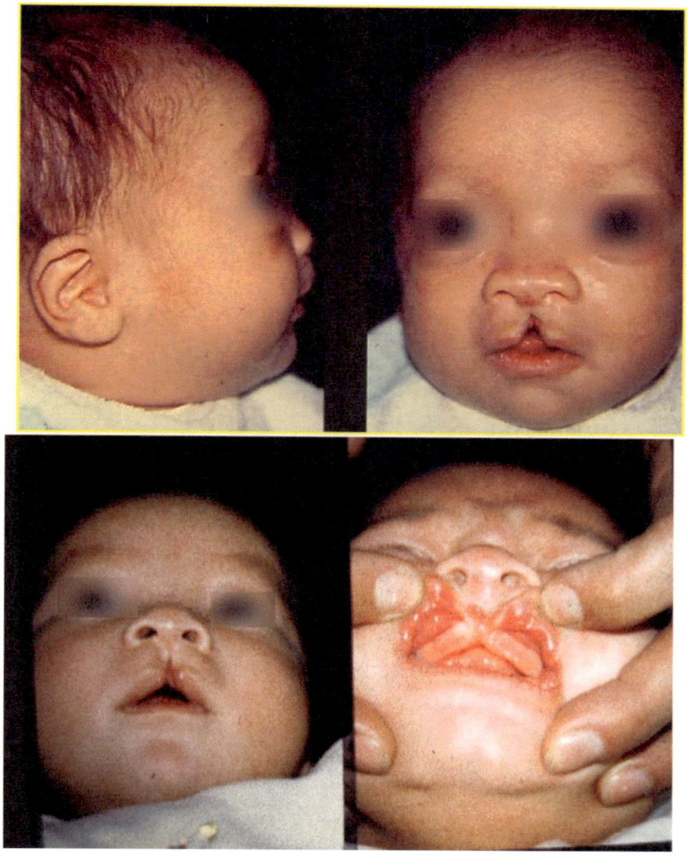

Figure 2.
Normo-hiperteleorbitism cases. Above the cleft involves all the upper lip and minor degree of hipertelorbitism is observed. Below other MCL patient with a double frenulum.

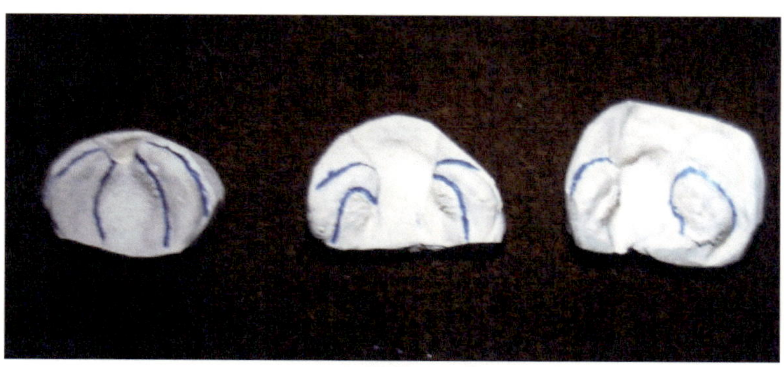

Figure 3.
Maxillary plaster models of 3 patients with Hypotelerbitism MCL in which a median maxillary defect of variable degree and absence of the premaxilla are observed.

Kawamoto added a sixth group patient with hypotelorism, flat nose, median cleft lips with normal brain morphology [13–15] and tried to complete the classification and put order. Indeed, this group denominated false median lip by Kawamoto corresponding to the Binderoid designed by Mulliken [16] or median false dysplasia of

Group	Morphology	Facial aspect	Brain
I	Cyclopia	Monophthalmia	Alobar
II	Etmocephaly	Extreme Hypotele and others	Alobar
III	Cebocephaly	Hypoteleorbitism and others	Alobar
IV	Hypoteleorbitism	Hypoteleorbtism and others	Alobar [usually]
V	Hypoteleorbitism	Hypoteleorbtism and others	Semilobar or lobar
VI*	Hypoteleorbitism	Hypoteleorbitism and others	Normal

Table 3.
Classification of holoprosencephaly [DeMyer].

**Kawamoto corresponds with Pseudomedian or False median cleft lip or Binderoid.*

Nordhoff [17]. It should be noted that they have MCL without or minimal malformations in the brain and survive but may look the same way as the Hypotelorbitism cases mentioned by DeMyer. They correspond to MCL with good prognosis. It is necessary to have a normal ultrasonic (US) or MRI exam for the right diagnosis. These clefts may be unilateral (**Figure 4**) or bilateral (**Figure 5**). In the first group, no Cupid's bow exists, and there are nasal and maxillary hypoplasia. In the bilateral form however, there is a tiny "pro-labium," some of them associated to cleft palate.

There are distinctive characteristics and prognosis between both main groups of DeMyer. **Table 4** shows a summary of the differences; 21 patients were of Hypoteleorbitism type and 34 patients had Normo-Hyperteleorbitism.

Notably, the group with Hypoteleorbitism is developed early in the third week, Carnegie state 8, and the size of the embryo is 0.4–2.5 mm. The Hyper-Normoteleorbitim was developed later, at 6- 8 weeks, the size of the embryo is 17 mm. Carnegie 17–20.

Wu [18] presents a classification of the MCL according to its extension of the cleft (**Figure 4**). When cleft involves only the vermilion is Number 1, Cleft 2 is committed vermilion and much of the lip (corresponds to the most common); type 3 extends to the columella, type 4 involves the nose. In type 5, there is a complete absence of the philtrum and premaxilla. In the revision, there are 8 cases of type 1, 23 cases of type 2, 2 cases of type 3, 1 case of type 4, and 21 cases of type 5. **Table 5** summarizes the distribution of the 34 patients.

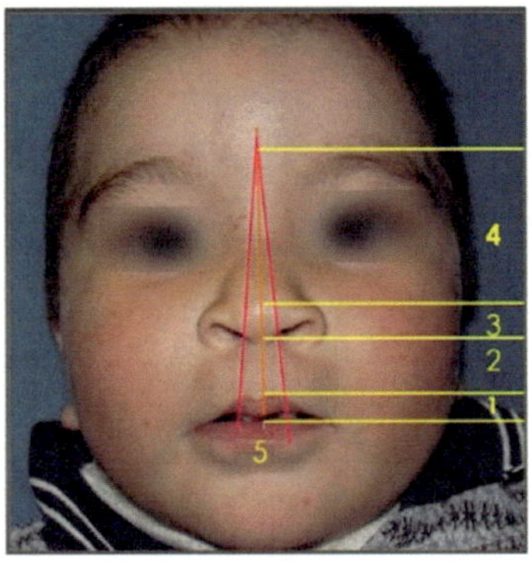

Figure 4.
Wu classification 5 groups depending on the extension of the cleft. The most frequent types are numbers 2 and 5.

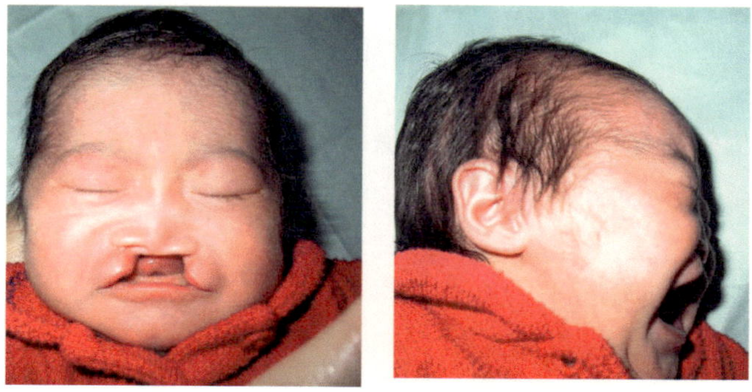

Figure 5.
A case of left cleft Type V Kawamoto or Binderoid (Mulliken). Observe the flat profile and wide right cleft.

	Hypoteleorbitism MCL	Normo or Hyper MCL
Median Cleft	+	+
Holoprosencephaly	+	—
Pro-Labium absence	+	—
Nose and Maxilla	Hypoplasia	Bifid or normal
Palate cleft	+	—
Brain abnormalities	+	—
Ocular malformations	+	—
Synophrys	+	—
Treatment	—	+
Vital prognosis	Poor	Excellent
Carnegie State	7–8	17–20
Size of the embryo	0.4–2.5 mm	17 mm

Table 4.
Differences between hypoteleorbitism MCL and Normo-Hyperteleorbitism MCL.

DeMayer Classification	Hypoteleorbitism	21 cases
	Hyperteleorbitism	34 cases
Wu Classification	Type I	8
	Type II	23
	Type III	2
	Type IV	2
	Type V	21

Table 5.
Distribution of 55 MCL cases.

Marie de Boutry [19, 20] is based in 14 patients, distinguished from 3 groups: Group I: Isolated MCL, Group II: MCL in association with craniofacial malformations, and Group III: MCL with extra facial malformations. Each group has different prognosis and specific treatment (**Figure 6**).

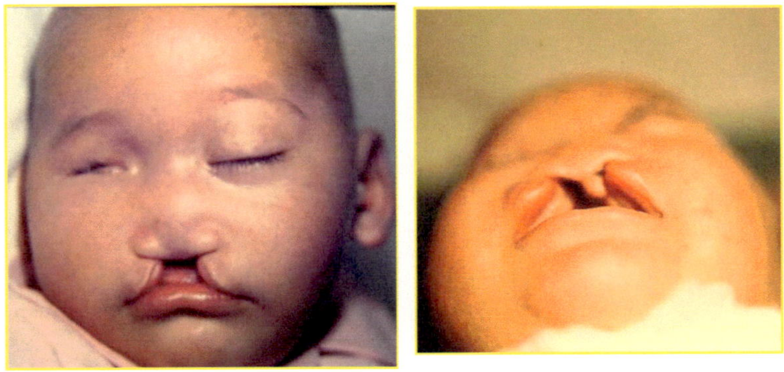

Figure 6.
Bilateral cleft Type VI Kawamoto with diminute prolabio, columella and flat nose, ultrasonography and MRI normal.

2.3 Associated syndromes

There are more than 200 syndromes associated with cleft lip and palate; however, few are related to MCL. We have observed two cases of the Ellis Van Creveld syndrome (**Figure 7**), Oro-Facial-Digital syndrome (**Figure 8**) and Pai syndrome [19, 20] 3 cases (**Figure 9**). Other associated syndromes are Thurton, Short rib polydactylies, Trisomy 21, and Frontonasal Dysplasia.

2.3.1 Management

Not all patients with MCL are amenable to surgical treatment. MCL with Hypoteleorbitism is in all cases out of surgical reach, because of severe intracranial malformations including HPE. Newborns with MCL and Alobar HPE (categories I, II, and III of DeMyer) rarely survive beyond 1 year of life, and these are not candidates for reconstruction. From our 21 cases with Hypotelorism, all died within a few days or months after they were born; one case survived painfully little more than 1 year. In **Figure 10**, you may observe five cases. These patients have an extreme flat nose, some of

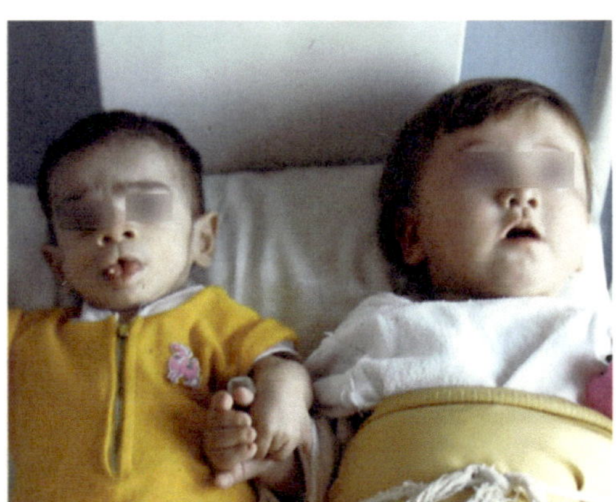

Figure 7.
Two patients with Ellis Van Creveld syndrome. A medial notch in the upper lip is observed and 6 normal fingers in each hand, cardiac malformations, and short stature.

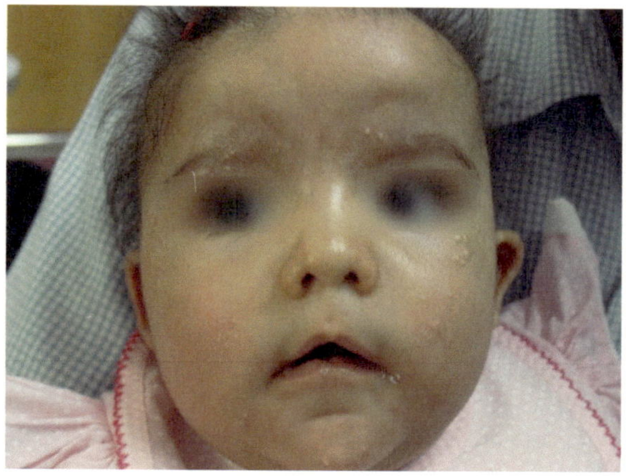

Figure 8.
Oro-Facial-Digital Syndrome is characterized by minor labial cleft, frenulated tongue, high arched or cleft palate, micrognathia palate, and hand anomalies.

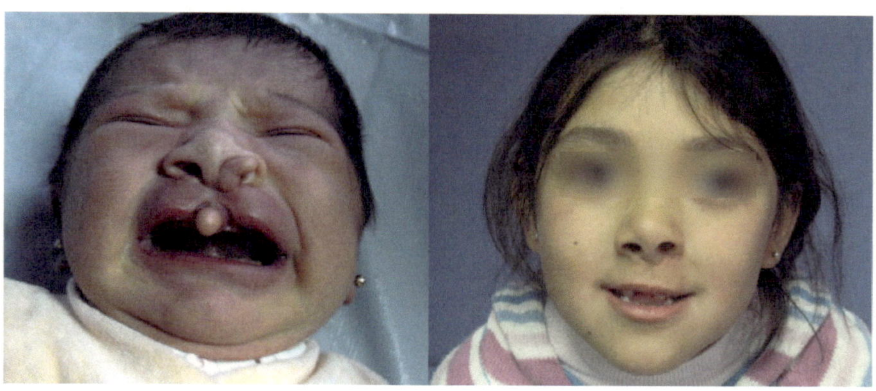

Figure 9.
A 3-month-old patient with Pai Syndrome and at 6 six years after the surgery. This syndrome includes an MCL, facial polypoid malformations, and lipoma in the corpus callus.

them with one single central nostril, absence of the premaxilla wide central palate cleft, poor living conditions, convulsions, difficulty for feeding, and low increase of weight.

Lately, some centers [21, 22] due to the progress in diagnosis, surgery, and postoperative care are treating selected cases with HPE; the surgical treatment is realized after 12 months of age; the mortality rate is 85% at 12 months of life. Indeed, the approach for patients with diverse types of HPE requires a multidisciplinary team including a pediatrician, neurologist, radiologist, genetician, and plastic surgeon. When a prenatal ultrasound (US) or Magnetic Resonance (MRI) exam shows HPE, the parents should receive the help and information of the team and a healthcare provider who is familiar with this condition, for planning the diverse treatment and alternatives, plus adequate parental counseling and genetic information. In many countries, it allows the interruption of pregnancy in cases of HPE. As soon as 9 weeks of pregnancy, the certain prenatal diagnosis of HPE with US and MRI is possible [23].

The subgroup VI without brain malformations or "binderoid" clefts is a good candidate for reconstruction, considering normality in terms of functionality and brain

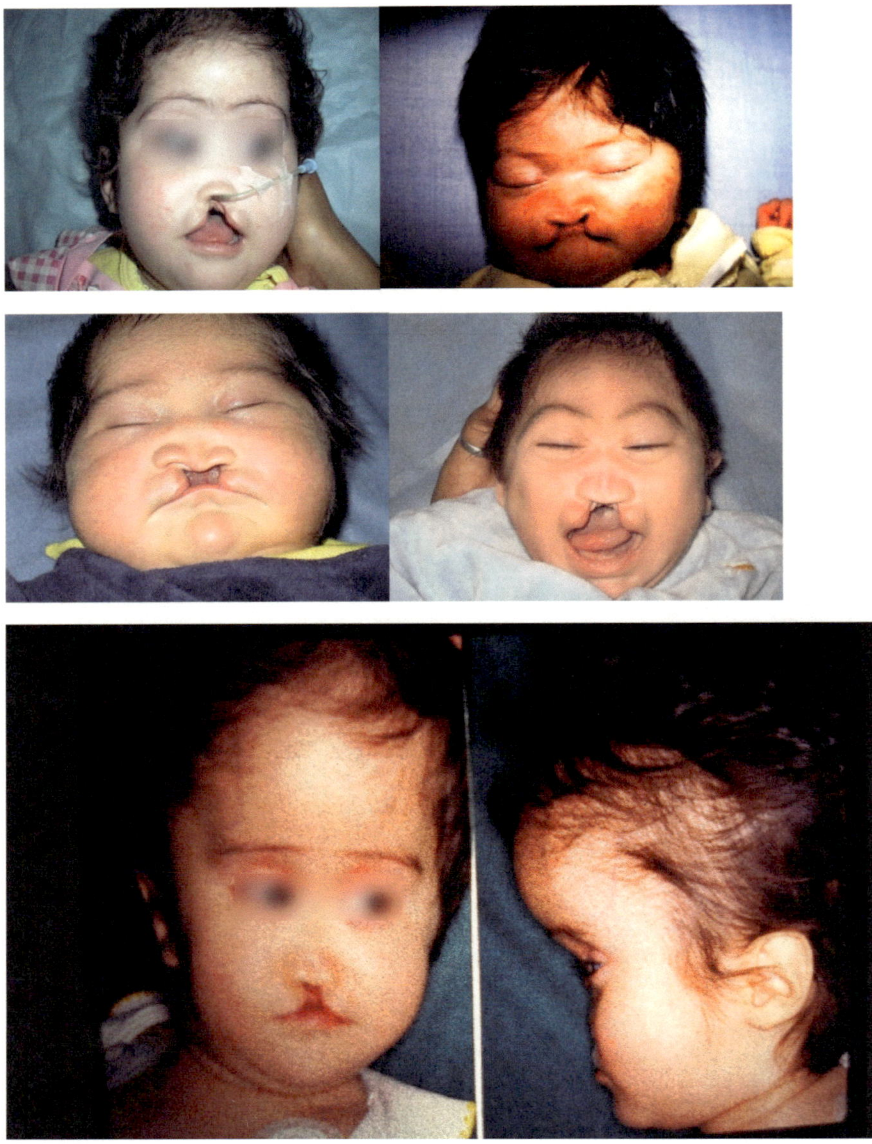

Figure 10.
Patients with MCL Demyer Hypotelorism type. There is a correlation between the severity of facial morphology and the development of the forebrain; looking the face you can guess how the brain is. No one survived.

anatomy. Given its good prognosis, patients are eligible for reconstructive surgery, may require complex treatments for management, including Abbe flap [24], nasal surgery, bone and cartilage grafts, maxillary distraction, and orthognathic surgery. Between ten cases of Binderoids clefts, 8 were unilateral and 2 bilateral. The surgery for unilateral cases was Rotation and Advancement technique or a primary Abbe flap, well tolerated in babies of 3 months of age; in bilateral, the closure was difficult because of the poor development of the prolabio. In the future is necessary perform nasal bone osteotomy and bone or cartilage graft to increase the projection of the nasal tip. In patients with type VI DeMyer, management may include maxillar surgery to correct the maxillary deficiency.

The surgical treatment in 34 patients with MC with Normal Hyperteleorbitism will depend on the type of deformity. The concepts of the surgical technique in the lip repair in MCL in these patients include excision of the cleft mar gins inverted V design, approach of the muscle plane, and alignment of the vermilion to restore the boundaries of the philtrum and the Cupid's bow.

The experience, particularly with Pseudomedian MCL management, in the primary operation the usual techniques of "rotation and advancement" or Abbe flap for uni lateral cases (**Figure 11**); in bilateral cases, both sides are operated at the same time when possible or with an Abbe flap technique (**Figure 12**).

In unilateral cases, the elements to properly reconstruct the Cupid's bow usually are not present, and therefore, we have used the Abbe flap as a primary procedure for the reconstruction of the philtrum. Later, costal cartilage grafts are placed in the premaxillary area and nose, which can be difficult because of the poor development of the nasal skin. The hypoplasia of the maxilla, which is progressive throughout the development, is an alternative that was used in the bone distraction with RED (Rigid External Distractor) system in 2 patients successfully, one 8-year-old male patient after an Abbe flap with 15 mm of sagittal discrepancy (achieving normal occlusion) (**Figure 13**) and another 18-year-old female patient after an Abbe flap, with 10 mm of sagittal discrepancy. **Figures 14–17** illustrate the different steps of the treatment from the newborn period to the final result at 25 years of age.

In MC type 1 of Wu, an inverted V incision will suffice to join the vermilion of the lip and rebuild the tubercle. If the double frenulum is present, it is removed and Z plasty may be done.

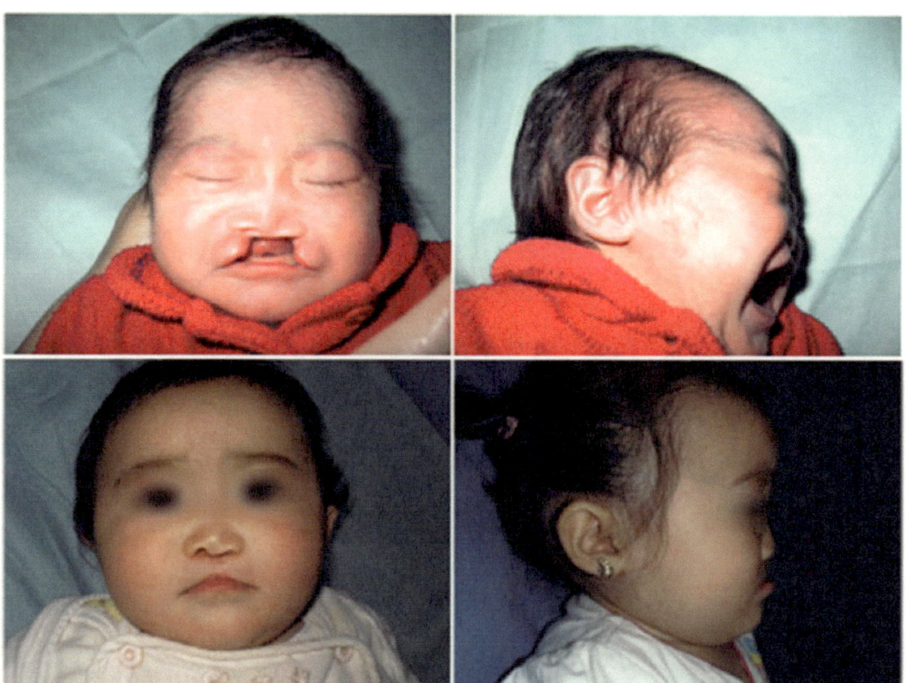

Figure 11.
Left pseudomedian cleft lip after Rotation and Advancement at 3 months of age.

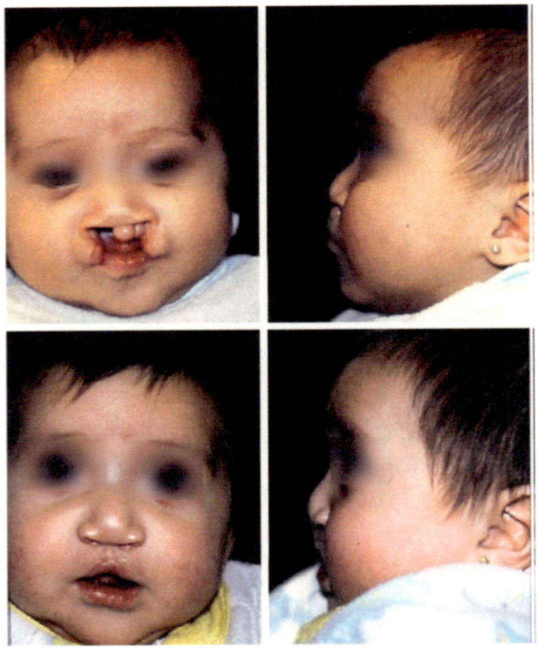

Figure 12.
Bilateral pseudomedian cleft lip, before and after reconstruction with Mulliken technique.

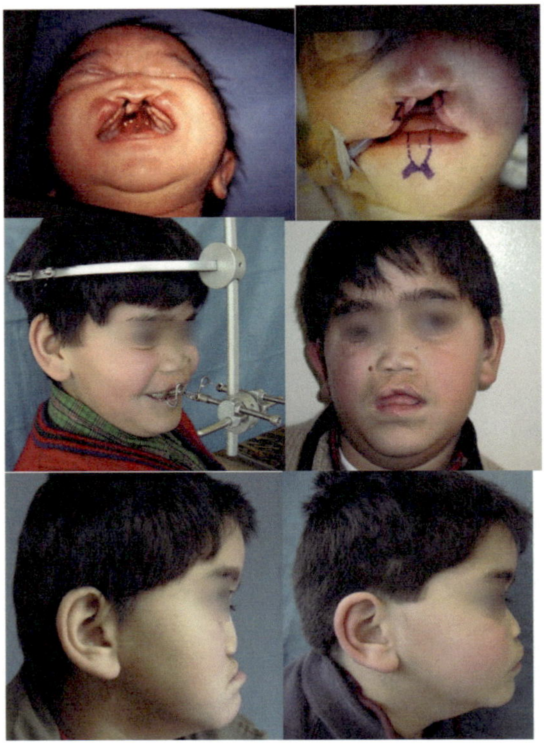

Figure 13.
Bilateral Pseudomedian case at various stages of treatment. Upper right Abbe flap design, middle left post op., and right with RED system. Above the profile shows an advancement of the maxilla was 8 mm.at 8 years of age.

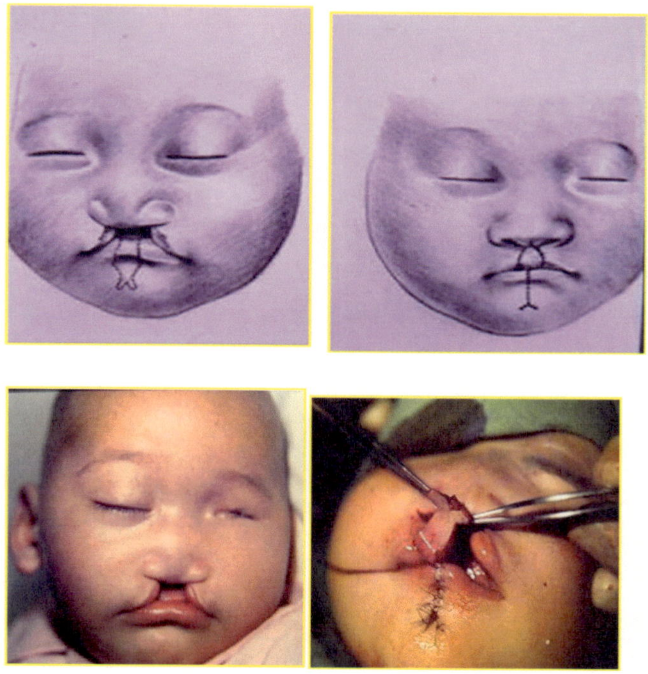

Figure 14.
Bilateral Psedomedio design of Abbe flap with two extensions for the reconstruction of the columella.

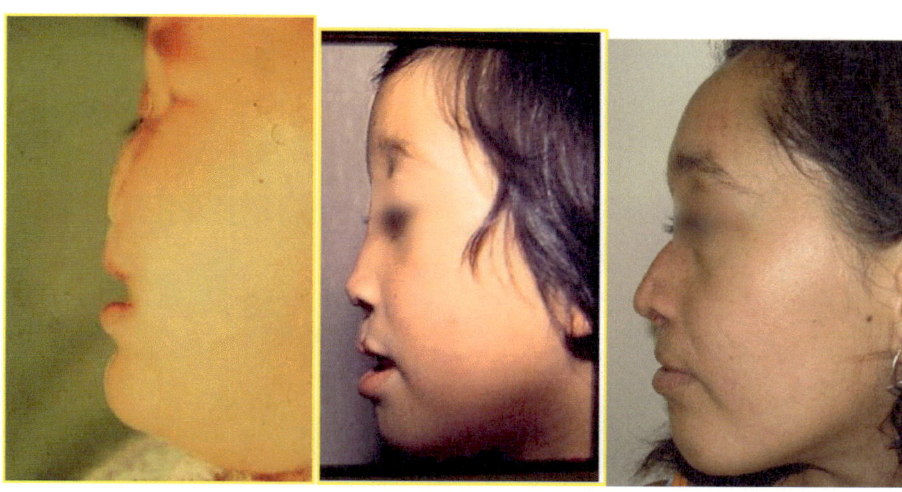

Figure 15.
Evolution of the profile after nasal bone and cartilage grafts plus maxillary distraction.

When the lip is more fully compromised (Wu type 2), an inverted V design is used; the orbicularis muscle is joint in the midline, and then, the skin is closed. The initial marking of the points must be done carefully in order to achieve a symmetrical Cupid's bow. The middle scars on the upper lip have a good outcome and are barely visible (**Figure 18**). Functional and esthetic anatomic correction was successfully achieved in each case without complication.

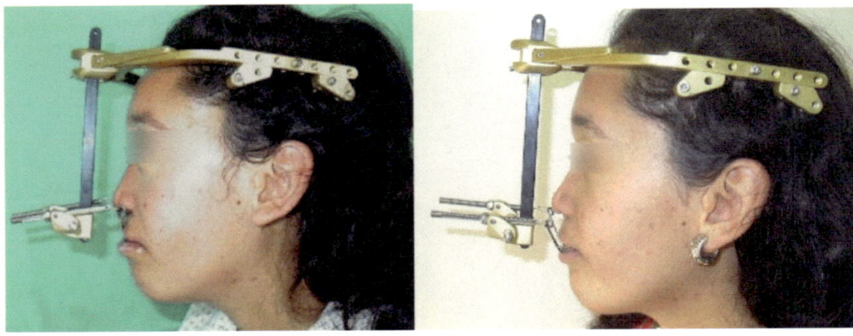

Figure 16.
Treatment with Rigid External Distraction; the improvement was10 mm of sagittal discrepancy.

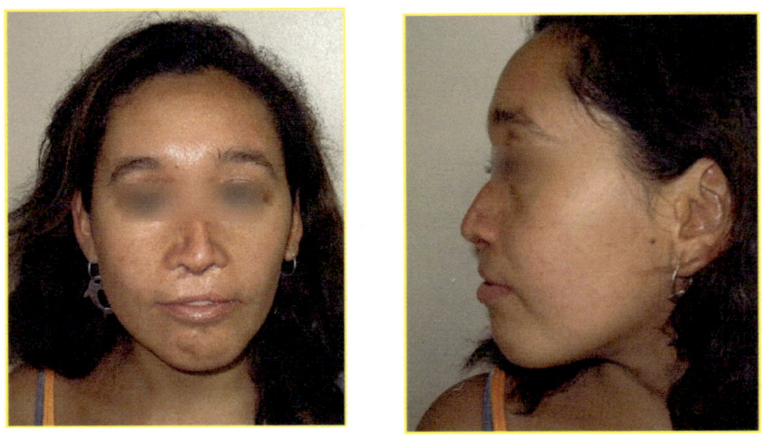

Figure 17.
Final result 25 years later.

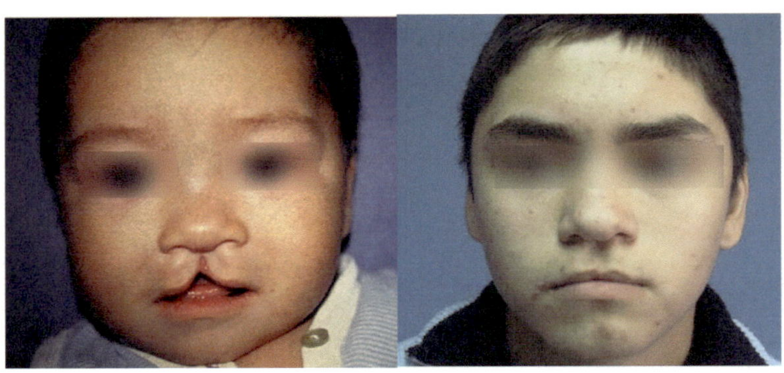

Figure 18.
Type 2 Wu MCL. Normoteleorbitism. The surgery was an inverted V-plasty at 3 months of age, result at 7 years; the central lip scar is not visible.

Type 3 Wu MC is treated the same way, but the incision is extended to the columella. It width is reduced by removing the excess skin, and the alar cartilages are bind in the midline. In **Figure 19**, the result of this procedure is demonstrated. We have treated MCL type 2 of Wu classification in 2 cases, in the context of Pai syndrome,

DOI: http://dx.doi.org/10.5772/intechopen.1012487

where the nasal mass compresses the nostril and causes a deformation of it. The pre- and postoperative results are in **Figures 9** and **20**. They will require additional surgery in the nostril to make the malformed nostril more symmetrical.

There are intricate cases requiring a "treatment team" with successive interventions carefully planned throughout their lives, repeated bone and cartilage grafts, bone distraction, dental pieces integration, and craniofacial and orthognathic surgery.

A unique complex case of MCL is in **Figure 21**, MCL associated to a medium degree of hyperteleorbotism, cleft palate, and an intrabuccal tumor. The tomographic scan shows two orifices, a normal one (Magnum) for the spinal cord and the other for a meningocele transcranial, intranasal, transpalatine, and intrabuccal. Complex neurosurgery removing the tumor and correction of the hypertelorism was done by Dr. Louis Morales in the Children Hospital of Salt Lake City. The senior author performed the treatment of the cleft lip and palate. He is now 24 years of age, with normal speech and looks, working as a medical technician. He required hormones during the growth process.

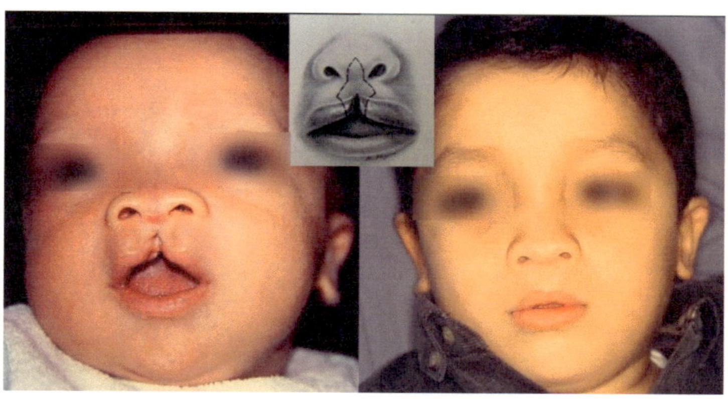

Figure 19.
Type 3 Wu MCL before and after surgery extended to the columella.

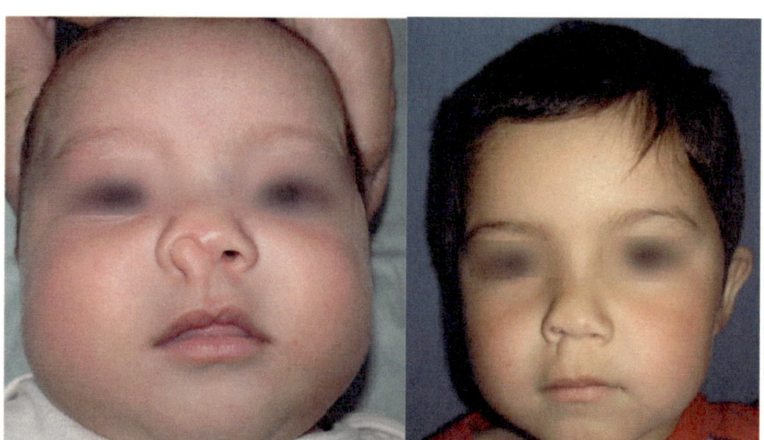

Figure 20.
Pai Syndrome, double frenulum, and midline premaxillary partial bone cleft, before and after reconstructive surgery.

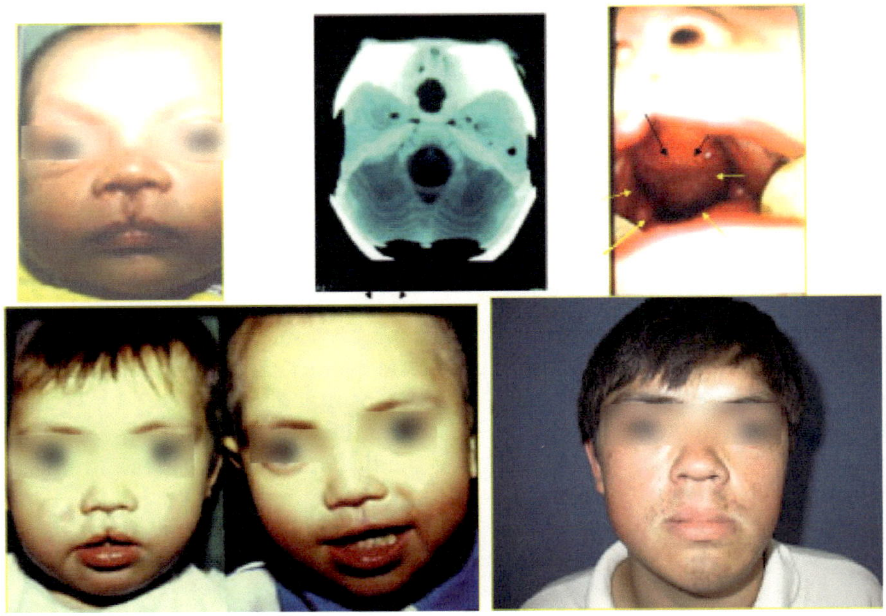

Figure 21.
Upper left: a Baby with MCL associated with cleft palate, hyperteleorbitism, and a meningocele transpalatine. The tomography in the center shows two orifices in base of the cranium; at right: a cleft palate and a large central meningocele. The result is after 4 surgeries and 20 years.

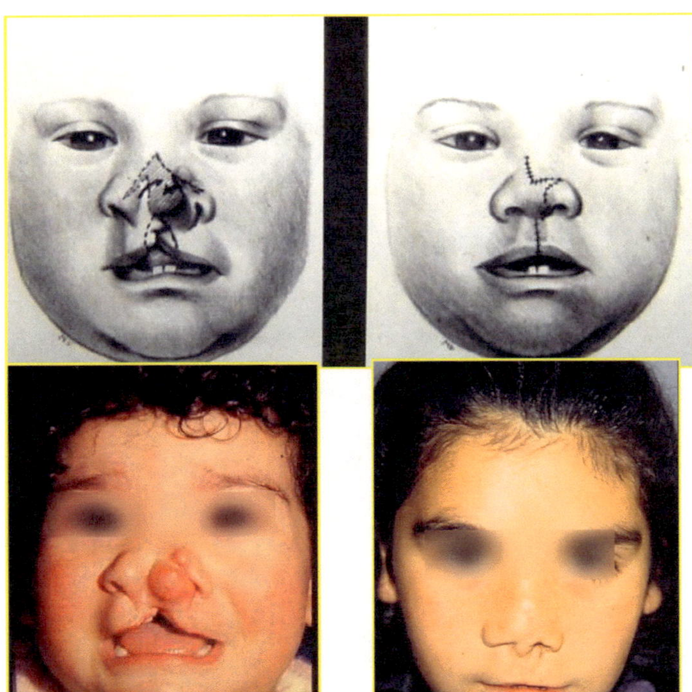

Figure 22.
Wu type 4 associated with PAE Syndrome. The nasal polypod structure was removed, and the lips and both nostrils were joined in the middle line. Result is after 7 years.

DOI: http://dx.doi.org/10.5772/intechopen.1012487

Figure 22 shows the only Wu type 4 associated with PAE Syndrome. The nasal polypod structure was removed, and the lip and both nostrils were joined in the middle line.

3. Conclusions

The median cleft corresponds to a rare disease, with low incidence in newborns and with great variability in its presentation, which limits the number of published articles. There are few casuistries with large numbers of patients, highlighting the casuistry of 55 cases.

The exact occurrence of a MCL is still unknown, although various causative factors have been published; outstanding are the theories of Carstens.

Several classifications of MCL have been established, the most used of which is DeMyer 1963, which has been modified in subsequent years so that you can establish a consistent behavior accord with the type of cleft.

Not all patients with MCL are amenable to treatment. MCL with Hypotelorism type I, II, and III is associated with HPE and does not require surgical treatment, because the life expectancy is less than 1 year. Genetic Council is recommended for the parents of babies with HPE. Type IV and type V may require management according to the degree of commitment and brain function, usually requiring limited corrective surgeries. The newborns with MCL with Hypotelorism type VI or "Binderoid" require comprehensive, surgical management, considering that their brain is normal in terms of development and functionality.

Patients with MCL Normo-Hypertelorism are clearly amenable to treatment, which depends on the severity, extent, and associated malformations that may arise and must be individualized for each case. Usually, the results are satisfactory.

The experience is shown with the results of treatment in hypo and normo-hiperteleorbitism and Binderoid type. Principles of treatment are explained. To achieve the best surgical result, cleft surgeons must adopt a comprehensive approach and meticulous preoperative planning for each individual patient. There is a wide variation of patients, sometime associated with other malformations. It is possible to use general principles of plastic and reconstructive surgery to obtain excellent results.

Acknowledgements

Thanks to Smile Train and Interplast for the help that we have received.

Conflict of interest

The authors declare no conflict of interest.

Author details

Luis Monasterio Aljaro[1*], Alison Ford Martinez de Pinillos[2] and Luis Fernando Monasterio Roman[2]

1 Fundación Gantz, Clínica Alemana, Santiago, Chile

2 Clínica Medicop, Santiago, Chile

*Address all correspondence to: eleemedr@hotmail.com

References

[1] Millard R, Williams S. Median cleft of the upper lip. Plastic and Reconstructive Surgery. 1968;**42**:4-14

[2] Tessier P. Anatomical classification facial, cranio-facial and latero-facial clefts. Journal of Maxillofacial Surgery. 1976;**4**:69-92

[3] Ortiz MF, Fuentes del Campo A, Dimoulus A. Nasal cleft. Annals of Plastic Surgery. 1987;**18**:377

[4] Adnan M, Faith BA, Tahir B, Merve Safa EA, Hasan BC. Median cleft lip. Journal of Craniofacial Surgery. 2023;**38**(8):780-781

[5] Dursy E. Zur Entwicklungsgeschichte des Kopfes des Mechen und der hoheren. Wirbeltheire. Tubigen: Verlag der H. Lauppschen-Buchhandlung; 1969

[6] Johnston MC. Morphogenesis and malformation of face and brain. Birth Defects. 1975;**11**:1

[7] Sulik KK. Craniofacial development. In: Turvey TA, Vig KWL, Fonseca RJ, editors. Facial Clefts and Craniosynostosis. Philadelphia: WB Saunders; 1986

[8] Carstens MH. Chapter 1. Mechanism of cleft palate developmental field analysis. In: Bennhum et al., editors. Cleft Lip and Palate Management. A Compressive Atlas. Hoboken. NJ: John Wiley & Sons; 2016

[9] Carstens M. Embryological Basis of Craniofacial Structures Developmental Anatomy, Evolutionary Design, and Clinical Applications. Heilderberg, Germany Springer; 2023

[10] Lavillaureix A, Rollier P, Kim A, Panasenkava V, De Tayrac M, Carré W, et al. DISP1 deficiency: Monoallelic and Biallelic variant causes a spectrum of midline craniofacial malformations. Genetics in Medicine. 2024;**26**:101126

[11] DeMyer W. The median cleft face syndrome. Differential diagnosis of cranial bifidum occultum, hypertelorism and median cleft nose, lip and palate. Neurology. 1967;**17**:961-971

[12] DeMyer W, Zeman W. Alobar holoprosencephaly (arrhinrncephaly) with median cleft lip and palate: Clinical electroencephalographic and nosologic considerations. Confinia Neurologica. 1963;**23**:1-36

[13] Kawamoto HK Jr. The kaleidoscopic world of rare craniofacial clefts: Order out of chaos (Tessier classification). Clinics in Plastic Surgery. 1976;**3**:529-572

[14] Kawamoto HK, Patel PK. Atypical facial clefts. In: Bentz M, editor. Pediatric Plastic Surgery. Stamford: Appleton and Lange; 1998

[15] Elias DL, Kawamoto HK, Wilson LF. Holoprosencephaly and midline facial anomalies: Redefining classification and management. Plastic and Reconstructive Surgery. 1992;**90**:951-958

[16] Mulliken JB, Burvin R, Padwa BL. Binderoid complete cleft lip/palate. Plastic and Reconstructive Surgery. 2003;**111**:1000-1010

[17] Noordhoff M, Huan C, Lo L. Medial facial dysplasia in unilateral and bilateral lip and palate: A subgroup of medial cerebrum facial malformations. Plastic and Reconstructive Surgery. 1993;**91**:996

[18] Wu R. Abstract. 8th International Congress on Cleft Lip/Palate and Related Craniofacial Anomalies. Singapore; 1997

[19] de Boutray M, Beziat J-L, Yachouh J, Bigorre M, Gleizal A, Captier G. The Journal of Craniofacial Surgery. 2016;**44**(6):664-671

[20] Pai GS, Levkoff AH, Leithiser RE Jr. Median cleft of the upper lip associated with lipomas of the central nervous system and cutaneus polyps. American Journal of Medical Genetics. 1987;**26**:921-924

[21] Butow KW, Zwahlen RA. Holoprosenecephay, with cleft: Data of 85 patients surgical treatment, and outcome: Part 2: Management, surgical treatment and unexpected aspect of holoprosencephaly cleft patients. Annals of Maxillofacial Surgery. 2019;**9**(1):146-151

[22] Morita N, Morita Y, Tanaka Y, Kimoto N, Ogawa H, Oomata T. Two cases of single-stage lip and nostril reconstruction in holoprosencephaly. International Journal of Oral and Maxillofacial Surgery. 2011;**40**(8):862-865

[23] Meagher S. Hui Alobar holoprosencephaly detected in a 9-week embrio. American Journal of Obstetrics and Gynecology. 2019;**221**(1):73-74

[24] Steinberg JP, Brady CM, Burstein FD. Primary Abbe flap for median cleft lip deformity: New trend an old concept. The Journal of Craniofacial Surgery. 2016;**27**(2):480-487

Chapter 4

Cleft Palate

Samar Mousa and Nitisha Narayan

Abstract

Cleft palate is one of the most common congenital facial differences. A thorough understanding of its embryological development, anatomical principles, and epidemiological patterns is essential for effective diagnosis and management. This chapter provides an insight into cleft palate, including its aetiology, incidence, classification, and the multidisciplinary approach required for optimal patient care. It describes in detail the evolution of cleft palate repair and current gold standard of care with relevant references and would be a useful read for any surgeon interested in cleft surgery, as well as plastics, maxillofacial and ENT trainees preparing for exams.

Keywords: cleft, palate, LAHSHAL, cleft pathway, palatoplasty, VPI

1. Introduction

The soft palate plays a key role in enabling speech, breathing, and swallowing by regulating the opening and closing of the connections between the oral, nasal, and pharyngeal cavities during each function. During swallowing, the soft palate becomes tense and aids in directing food down the digestive tract. It then elevates to block access to the nasal cavity, preventing food from entering the nasal passages. While breathing through the nose, the soft palate lowers and makes contact with the base of the tongue, ensuring that food does not enter the oropharynx and interfere with the flow of exhaled air [1].

In speech, the soft palate elevates and becomes tense. The back of the tongue presses against it to produce velar consonants such as [k], [g], and [ŋ] in English. This movement must close off the nasal cavity to avoid air escaping through the nose, which would result in nasal-sounding speech. Developmental issues with the palate are common and can lead to conditions such as cleft lip or cleft palate. These congenital abnormalities may cause significant challenges with feeding, speech, and recurrent infections in affected infants [1].

A cleft palate is a very common congenital craniofacial defect defined by an opening or gap in the mouth's roof caused by inadequate fusion of the palatal tissues during embryological development. Newborns with a cleft palate frequently struggle with feeding and achieving an effective latch, which can lead to weariness from the additional effort necessary during feeding. The cleft interferes with the natural separation between the nasal and oral chambers, resulting in nasal regurgitation of food and drink. Furthermore, the improper attachment and direction of the muscle influences speech development. The improper attachment of the muscles and its capacity to vent the auditory tube can lead to recurrent ear infections and conductive hearing loss [2]. To fully appreciate the clinical implications of cleft palate and the principles guiding its management, it is essential first to develop a sound understanding of the normal anatomy and embryological formation of the palate.

2. Anatomy and embryology

The palate constitutes the roof of the mouth, separating the oral and nasal cavities (**Figure 1**). It is separated into two sections: an anterior, static, hard bony segment and a posterior, moveable soft palate without bony features. The hard palate (**Figure 2**) accounts for approximately two-thirds of the total surface area of the palate, and its underlying bony structure is created by the maxillary palatine processes and the palatine bones' horizontal plates. The palatine processes of the maxilla account for the majority of the hard palate anteriorly, stretching between the two sides of the maxillary dental arch. They connect posteriorly to the palatine bones' horizontal plates and fuse along the midline. The hard palate also has three foramina, or canals, which serve as conduits for vital neurovascular systems that supply the oral cavity. The "incisive canal", "greater palatine foramen", and "lesser palatine foramen" serve as important anatomical indicators (**Table 1**) [8].

The soft palate is composed of muscle fibres encased in mucous membrane and plays an important role in breathing and swallowing, comprising five major muscles (**Figure 3**).

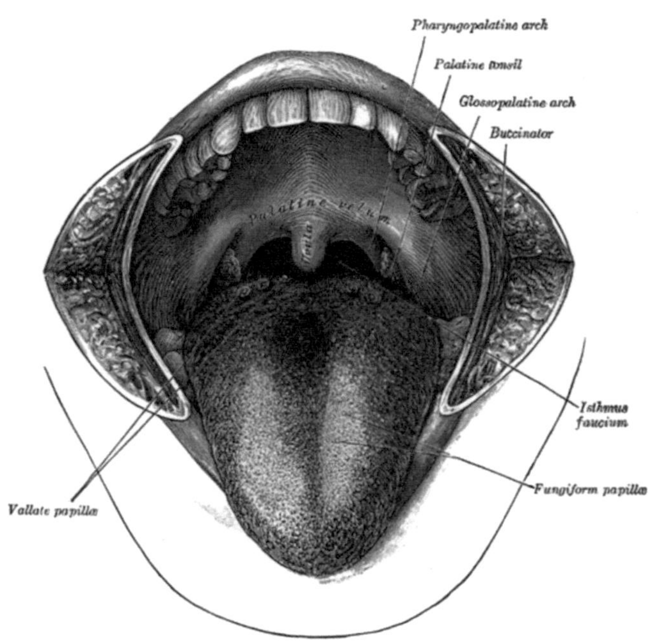

Figure 1.
Anatomy of the human palate [3]. This work is in the public domain in the United States because it was published (or registered with the U.S. Copyright Office) before January 1, 1930.

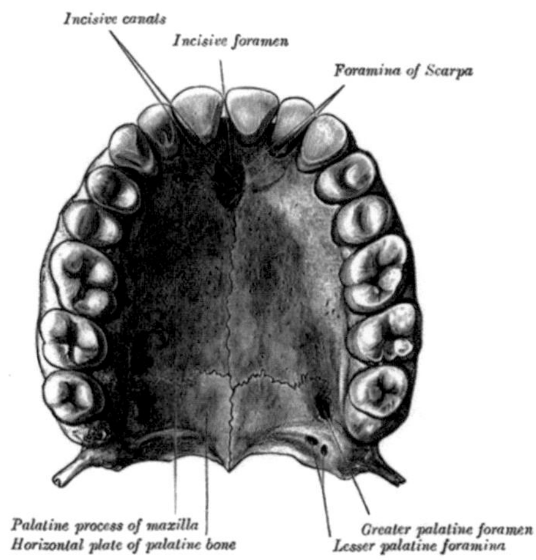

Figure 2.
The bony palate and alveolar arch [4]. This work is in the public domain in the United States because it was published (or registered with the U.S. Copyright Office) before January 1, 1930.

Veau Classification [5]	
I	Soft palate only
II	Hard and soft palate up to the incisive foramen
III	Unilateral cleft of the soft/hard palate, lip, and alveolus
IV	Bilateral cleft of the soft/hard palate, lip, and alveolus
Kernahan and Stark [6]	
1	Anterior to the incisive foramen
2	Posterior to the incisive foramen
3	Spanning both regions
American Cleft Palate Craniofacial Association (ACPA) Classification [7]	
1	Prepalate (lip, alveolus, primary palate): cheiloschisis, alveoloschisis, cheiloalveoloschisis,
2	Palate (secondary palate): uranoschisis, staphyloschisis, uranostaphyloschisis
3	Combined clefts: alveolocheilopalatoschisis
4	Other facial clefts (e.g., oro-ocular, oroaural)

Table 1.
Veau, Kernahan, and Stark and ACPA classification of cleft palate.

- The “Levator veli palatini muscle” lifts the soft palate and aids in swallowing.
- The “Musculus uvulae muscle” shortens the uvula.
- The “Palatoglossus muscle” pushes the soft palate towards the tongue, facilitating swallowing.
- The “palatopharyngeus muscle” helps with breathing by tensing the soft palate

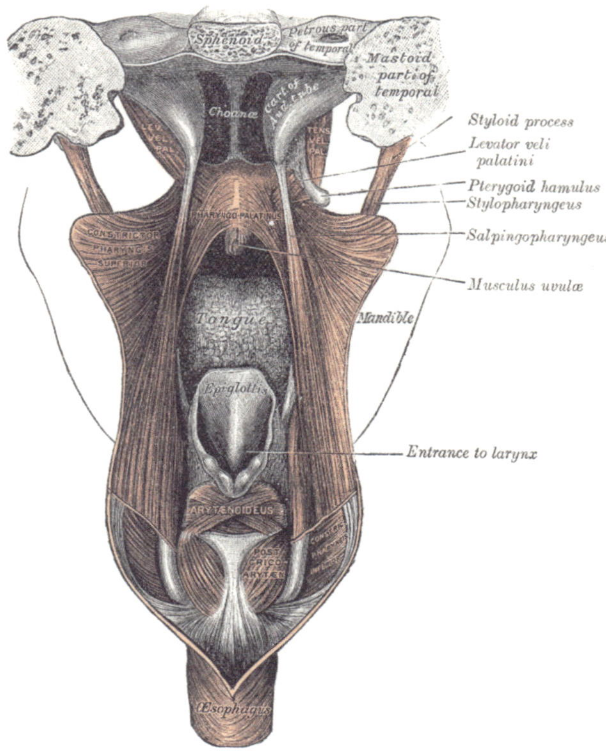

Figure 3.
Anatomy of the palatine muscles [9]. This work is in the public domain in the United States because it was published (or registered with the U.S. Copyright Office) before January 1, 1930.

- and pulling the pharynx anteriorly.
- The "tensor veli palatini muscle" helps with swallowing by tensing the soft palate [8].

The soft palate is joined to the tongue and the pharynx by two arches: palatoglossal and palatopharyngeal (**Figure 3**). The palatine tonsils are situated between these arches in the tonsillar fossa of the oropharynx. During swallowing, the levator veli palatini raises the soft palate, bringing it into contact with the posterior pharyngeal wall and essentially closing the airway and nasal passages. This produces a vacuum in the oral cavity, keeping food from entering the respiratory tract. The elevated soft palate mechanically closes the airway when swallowing, causing breathing to be halted for a brief period [10, 11].

2.1 Blood supply and lymphatics

The greater palatine arteries supply the palate by travelling anteriorly from the greater palatine foramen. They are the principal artery supply for the palate. An anastomosis connects the ascending and lesser palatine arteries, allowing for collateral circulation. Both the greater and lesser palatine arteries are branches of the maxillary artery, which is derived from the external carotid artery. The ascending palatine artery is a branch of the facial artery that originates from the external carotid artery. Venous drainage from the palate leads to the pterygoid venous plexus. Lymphatic drainage from the soft palate enters the subdigastric and/or lateral pharyngeal lymph nodes [12, 13].

2.2 Nerve supply

With the exception of the tensor veli palatini muscle, all palatal muscles are innervated by fibres of the pharyngeal plexus, which originates from the vagus nerve. The medial pterygoid nerve, which is a branch of the trigeminal nerve, innervates the tensor veli palatini muscle. The trigeminal nerve's maxillary branch provides sensory innervation to the palate. The maxillary division produces a number of sensory branches that serve the midface region, including the nasopalatine, larger palatine, lesser palatine, superior alveolar, middle meningeal, infraorbital, zygomatic, inferior palpebral, superior labial, and pharyngeal nerves. The greater palatine nerve exits from its canal through the greater palatine foramen and travels anteriorly along the roof of the palate, innervating the gingivae and mucosa of the hard palate and communicating with the nasopalatine nerve. The lesser palatine nerve arises from the lesser palatine foramen and runs alongside the greater palatine nerve, providing sensory innervation to the tonsils, uvula, and soft palate [14].

2.3 Embryology

During early embryonic development, the nasal and oral chambers are continuous because no anatomical structure divides them. As development *progresses*, the construction of the palate divides these two chambers. The primary palate is formed by the sixth week of gestation, followed by the secondary palate between the sixth and eighth weeks (**Figure 4**). During the sixth week, the medial nasal and maxillary processes fuse, forming the primary palate, which contains the alveolar arch and coincides with external face development [16–18].

The secondary palate, which includes both the hard and soft palates, develops from palatal shelves that emerge vertically from the medial walls of the maxillary processes, lateral to the tongue and posterior to the primary palate. Around the eighth week of gestation, these ledges realign horizontally above the tongue as the jaw expands and the tongue descends. Fusion starts anteriorly, just beyond the major palate, and moves posteriorly in a "zipper-like" pattern [19].

When the palatal shelves meet at the midline, the medial edge epithelium contacts and fuses, generating a midline epithelial seam. This seam eventually degenerates, allowing mesenchymal continuity throughout the palate [20]. The mesenchyme then separates into bone within the hard palate and soft tissue within the soft palate [21]. Failure of this fusion process leads in a cleft palate, which is caused by aberrant development of the palate or surrounding structures during gestation [2].

Clefting disturbs the palatal muscles' natural anatomical alignment, causing them to shift to a more sagittal orientation with insertion along the hard palate's posterior edge. This change disrupts normal muscular activity, altering speech resonance and the capacity to make plosive sounds [22].

The cleft line usually starts on the lateral part of the upper lip and runs through the philtrum to the alveolus, notably between the lateral incisor and the canine, then down the sutura incisiva to the foramen incisivum. Clefting prior to the incisive

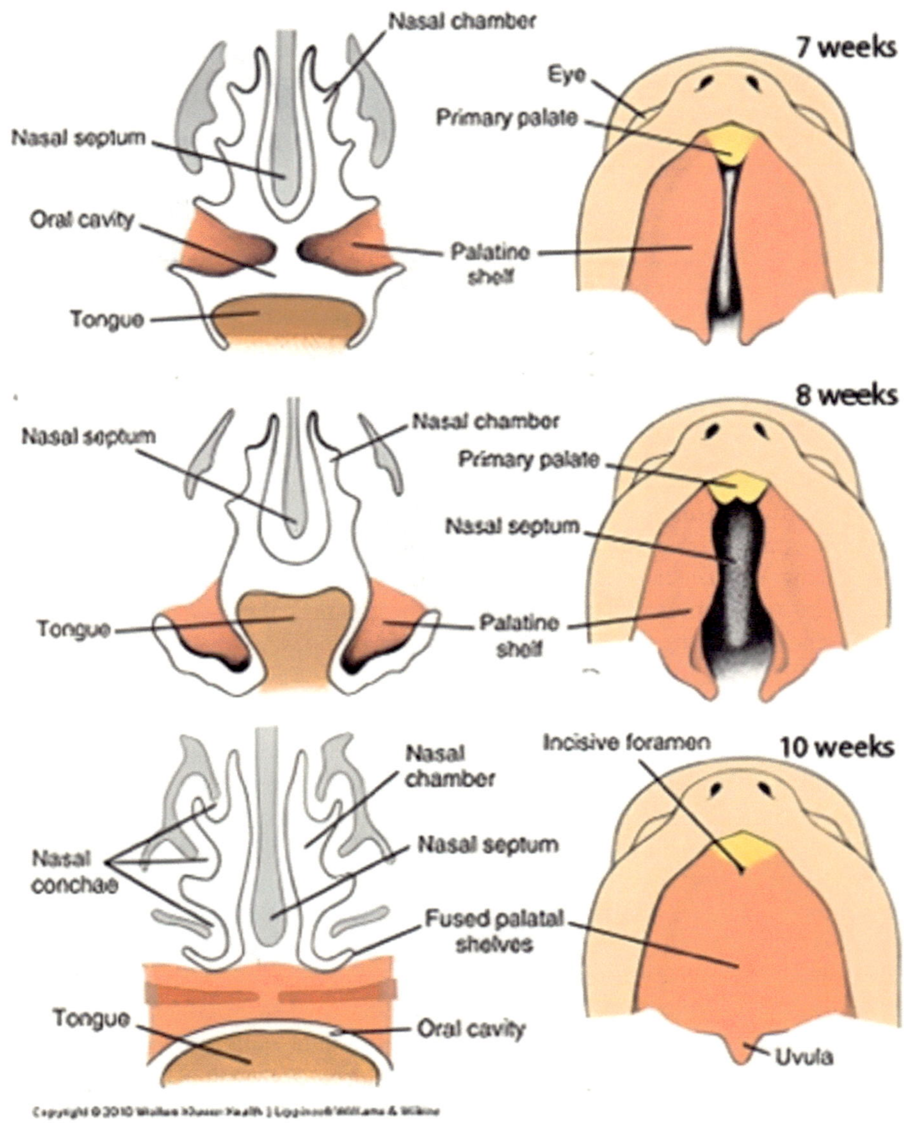

Figure 4.
The development of the palate from 7 to 10 weeks of gestation showing the reorientation of the palatal shelves. Ref. [15].

foramen, involving the lip and alveolus, is referred to as a primary palate cleft, whereas clefting posterior to the incisive foramen is classed as a secondary palate cleft (**Figure 5**). A complete cleft palate consists of a cleft in the hard palate, soft palate, and uvula [24].

In many cases, the hard palate cleft is covered by healthy mucosa and extends into the soft palate, resulting in a submucous cleft palate. This disease is distinguished by a midline palatal lucency, known as the "zona pellucida," which is usually evident due to the separation of the levator muscles, as well as a notch in the posterior hard palate, indicating the lack of the posterior nasal spine. Patients may also exhibit a bifid uvula [24]. Cleft palates often present in two distinct shapes: a V-shaped cleft, most

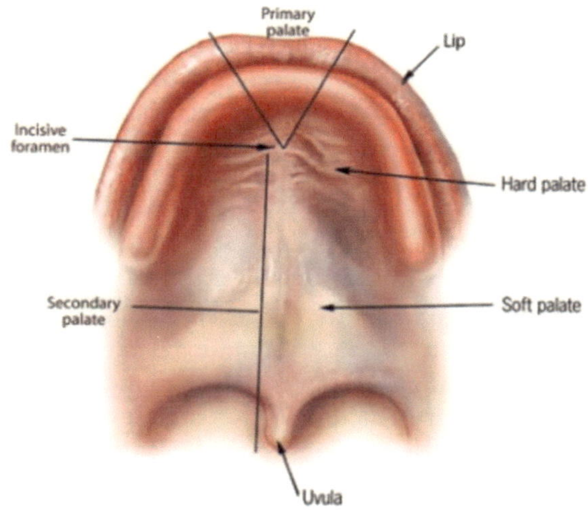

Figure 5.
The primary and secondary palate separated by the incisive foramen [23].

commonly observed in isolated cases, and a U-shaped cleft, which is more frequently connected with the Robin sequence and syndromic variants [25].

3. Epidemiology

3.1 Incidence

Cleft lip and palate are the most frequent craniofacial birth defects [22]. Despite its importance, current published data on the demographics of cleft palate are few and vary widely in terms of reported frequency and demographics [26]. According to the World Health Organisation (WHO), cleft lip and palate diagnosis rates vary by geography and ethnicity, with Asian and Latino populations having the highest prevalence, followed by certain Native American groups, and Black populations having the lowest rates [27–29].

Salari et al.'s [30] evaluation of 57 research involving 17,907,569 individuals discovered that the global prevalence of cleft palate was 0.33 per 1000 live births (95% CI: 0.28–0.38). Based on 55 studies comprising 17,894,673 individuals, the cumulative prevalence of cleft lip and palate was reported to be 0.45 per 1000 live births (95% CI: 0.38–0.52) [30].

According to the CRANE (Cleft Registry and Audit NEtwork) 2024 Annual Report, cleft lip and/or palate affects roughly one out of every 660 live births in the United Kingdom, including all types of orofacial clefts [31]. While the study does not define the frequency of cleft palate alone, prior CRANE data from 2020 showed that isolated cleft palate occurs at a rate of about 15 per 10,000 live births in England, Wales, and Northern Ireland. Furthermore, females were more likely to have clefts (17 per 10,000 female live births) than males (13 per 10,000 male live births) [32].

Cleft palate can occur as an isolated condition or alongside cleft lip and other orofacial clefts, and it is associated with over 150 known syndromes, such as Stickler syndrome, Down syndrome, Treacher Collins syndrome, Beckwith-Wiedemann syndrome, craniosynostosis syndromes, and Pierre Robin sequence [33, 34]. Children with cleft palate, particularly those with a syndromic diagnosis, often present with additional airway anomalies that require careful evaluation during the perioperative period. The term "palatal shelf hypoplasia" describes the underdevelopment of the palatal structures that results in a cleft palate. This condition is commonly linked to syndromes like Pierre Robin sequence and may necessitate staged surgical repair due to the presence of a wide palatal gap [35].

3.2 Aetiology

Several risk factors have been found for the development of orofacial clefting. These include genetic predisposition and environmental exposure. Certain drugs, including phenytoin, sodium valproate, topiramate, and methotrexate, have also been linked to an increased risk. Lifestyle factors such as smoking, tobacco use, and alcohol use have been linked to an elevated risk. Furthermore, maternal folate deficiency, maternal obesity, and pre-existing diabetes—rather than gestational diabetes—have been identified as significant causes. If there is a family history of cleft lip or palate in parents or siblings, the likelihood of having another child with a cleft increases [27, 28].

4. Classification

The understanding and classification of cleft lip and palate have evolved greatly throughout time, with early references referring to the disorder as "harelip" because of its similarity to a hare's mouth. Davis and Ritchie explicitly rejected this term at the 1922 American Medical Association convention, instead advocating for the more clinical term "congenital cleft of the lip" [36, 37]. Several classification schemes have since been presented, but no single approach has gained widespread support [38]. Veau proposed a basic, morphology-based system with four types, ranging from isolated soft palate clefts to complete bilateral clefts of the lip, alveolus, and palate [5]. Kernahan and Stark (1958) established a system focused on the incisive foramen that classified clefts as anterior, posterior, or crossing both regions, as well as considering laterality and severity [6]. Harkins et al. classified clefts according to the American Cleft Palate-Craniofacial Association (ACPA) using anatomical regions—prepalate, palate, and combined clefts—and included technical terms such as cheiloschisis and uranoschisis, as well as laterality, severity, and vomer involvement [7].

Kernahan's Striped-Y classification [39] evolved from his previous approach, providing a simplified visual representation (**Figure 6**) for clinical application. Later enhancements by Elsahy [40] and Millard [41] increased its utility. In 1981, the ACPA accepted both this approach and its 1962 classification for their clarity and embryological relevance, preferring the phrases "primary/secondary palate" or "prepalate/palate" over "anterior/posterior palate," and recommending grouping median cleft lip with orofacial clefts [38]. The LAHSHAL system [42], which is based on Kernahan and Stark's [6] symbolic classification, uses an acronym to represent cleft involvement in the Lip, Alveolus, Hard palate, and Soft palate (**Figure 6**). From the patient's right to left, it employs capital letters for entire clefts, lowercase for incomplete ones, an asterisk (*) for microforms, a dot (•) for unaffected areas, and a plus (+) to signify Simonart's band. A case with complete bilateral cleft lip, incomplete alveolar clefts, and an incomplete soft palate cleft is denoted as "La•s•aL".

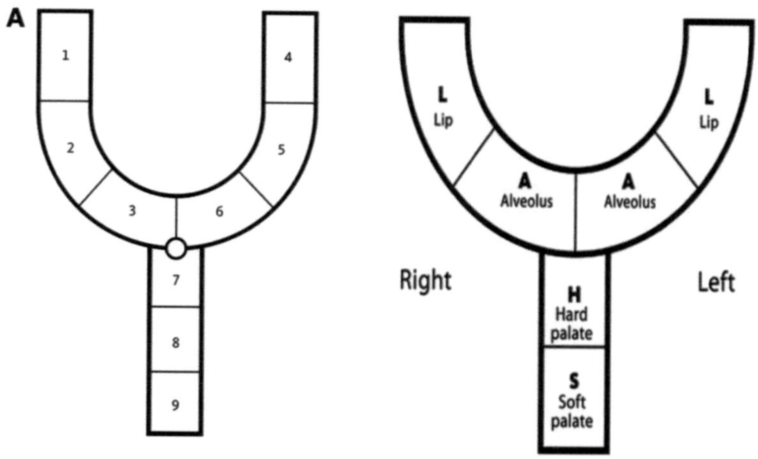

Figure 6.
The "striped-Y" classification system developed by Kernahan that divides the primary and secondary palate by the incisive foramen. Available via licence: CC BY-NC-ND 4.0 and diagrammatic representation of the LAHSHAL classification system of cleft lip and palate. Available via licence: CC BY-NC-ND 4.0.

While the ICD-10 system was designed primarily for disease registration, it is also widely used in epidemiology, global disease burden tracking, and healthcare reimbursement [43–46]. Despite limits in precision and comprehensiveness [38], it has achieved universal acceptance as a result of required usage by health registries and insurers in Europe and North America. A global survey by Houkes et al. [47] indicated that ICD-10 (35.5%) was the most often used categorisation, followed by LAHSHAL (34%), Veau (32.5%), Striped-Y (22.8%), and ACPA (21.3%), demonstrating the lack of a universally approved system [46]. In the United Kingdom, LAHSHAL is the chosen system for national cleft registry reporting [31].

5. Assessment

5.1 History

A complete history should begin with information about the prenatal period, birth, and developmental milestones. A complete medical history is required, which should include any syndromic or medical diagnoses, a history of ear infections or middle ear effusions, interventions for hearing loss (whether temporary or permanent), including the use of grommets, as well as known allergies and persistent nasal congestion. Neurological diseases or injuries should be documented, as well as current medications and any previous or ongoing feeding, swallowing, nasal regurgitation, nasal breathing, or snoring issues. The background history should also include any family history of cleft palate, velopharyngeal dysfunction (VPD), resonance disorders, or speech and language problems. A complete surgical history is necessary, describing any cleft lip and/or palate procedures, including dates and patient age at the time of surgery, as well as other pertinent operations such as tonsillectomy, adenoidectomy, or frenectomy. Finally, any problems about feeding, breathing, snoring, hearing, or vision should be documented, as well as the family's assessment of the child's general quality of life [48].

5.2 Examination

A visual inspection of the hard and soft palates should be performed within the first 24 hours of life, using a torch and tongue depressor to evaluate the whole length of the palate from the gums to the uvula [49]. If the initial inspection is incomplete, a second attempt should be performed within the next 24 hours, with parents notified. This evaluation should also look at craniofacial structures (face, nose, eyes, ears, skull, profile) for symmetry and proportion, as well as oral structures (lips, jaw, tongue, velum) for movement, strength, and abnormalities like clefts, fistulas, macroglossia, ankyloglossia, bifid uvula, or a narrow maxilla. Observations should include the link between the length of the soft palate and the oropharyngeal depth, as well as the size of the tonsils, because they affect speech resonance and airway function. To reduce ambiguity, it is advised that findings be documented using a visual diagram [50].

Audiological testing is an essential component of early evaluation. It should involve otoscopic examination, immittance testing, pure-tone air and bone conduction testing, otoacoustic emissions as needed, and speech threshold and discrimination testing based on the child's age and ability [48]. Because neonates with cleft palate frequently fail the initial hearing screening due to middle ear effusions, a thorough audiology evaluation is essential. Eustachian tube dysfunction is prevalent, increasing the risk of recurrent otitis media and conductive hearing loss [37]. Feeding and swallowing examinations should focus on feeding habits, particularly indicators of nasal regurgitation. When appropriate, objective examinations such as fibre-optic endoscopic evaluation of swallowing (FEES) and videofluoroscopic swallowing study (VFSS) should be used. These evaluations must take into account the child's age, developmental condition, and surgical history, with suitable modifications such as specialist bottles and teats [48].

6. Management

The management of cleft palate necessitates a collaborative effort across various disciplines. This team usually consists of specialists in plastic surgery, oral and maxillofacial surgery, dentistry, orthodontics, otolaryngology, neurology, genetics, nutrition, speech therapy, and child development. Parents of babies diagnosed with cleft lip and palate antenatally or at birth can expect the cleft team to begin consultations immediately after delivery, with continued treatment extending into adulthood [37]. Over the last two decades, significant efforts have been undertaken worldwide to standardise and streamline the perioperative management of patients with cleft palate, with various degrees of success in Europe, the United Kingdom, and North America. Nonetheless, significant variance exists between centres, with decisions about surgical repair and perioperative treatment heavily influenced by the surgeon's specific knowledge, training, and experience [22].

In the United States, a structured treatment pathway begins in the antenatal and perinatal periods with team introduction, genetic counselling, and feeding support, followed by staged interventions: cleft lip repair (1–3 months), palate repair (9–12 months), speech and hearing monitoring, dental and orthodontic management, alveolar bone grafting, and potential surgeries such as rhinoplasty and orthognathic procedures, extending into early adulthood with attention to dental implantation and family planning counselling [51].

In the United Kingdom, cleft lip (with or without cleft palate) is regularly identified prenatally with 2D ultrasound between 20 and 22 weeks, but isolated cleft palate is more difficult to detect without advanced imaging such as 3D ultrasound or MRI [52–57]. Following birth, a cleft nurse expert provides feeding assistance within 24 hours [58]. Lip restoration usually takes 3–6 months, followed by soft palate repair between 9 and 13 months to aid speech development [59–61]. Speech monitoring, dental help, and regular multidisciplinary examinations at national audit clinics at the ages of 5, 10, 15, and 20 are all part of ongoing care [57, 62–64]. During childhood and adolescence, patients receive dental and orthodontic care, including planning for alveolar bone transplantation prior to permanent canine eruption [60, 61]. Some may require additional speech surgery or orthognathic treatments to address skeletal abnormalities [60, 62]. Individuals who are discharged in early adulthood might return to the cleft service if they want restorative dental care or genetic counselling while having a family (**Figure 7**) [65].

The CLP Registry is Sweden's National Quality Registry that monitors children and adolescents with cleft lip and/or palate. It was launched in 1999 at Sweden's six CLP centres to reduce treatment variability. All children with CLP are recruited and tracked from birth to adulthood, with treatment and outcome data obtained at crucial periods (5, 10, 16, and 19). While treatment techniques vary slightly between facilities, all execute lip-nose repair within 3–6 months, with varying approaches to palatal surgery and standardised secondary bone grafting within 7–11 years. The registry allows for early diagnosis of unsatisfactory results and facilitates rapid improvements in care [66].

In Taiwan, craniofacial anomaly treatment begins within the first week of life with presurgical orthopaedics and nasoalveolar moulding (NAM). Surgical treatment comprises one-stage lip repair at 3 months for moderate instances or a two-stage technique for larger clefts, as well as nose reconstruction. Palatoplasty is performed at 12 months with grommet tube insertion. Speech examination begins at 2.5 years, and velopharyngeal insufficiency (VPI) is diagnosed and treated after age 4. Alveolar bone grafting (ABG) is performed prior to canine eruption, generally in conjunction with VPI surgery, and is followed by comprehensive orthodontics once the dentition

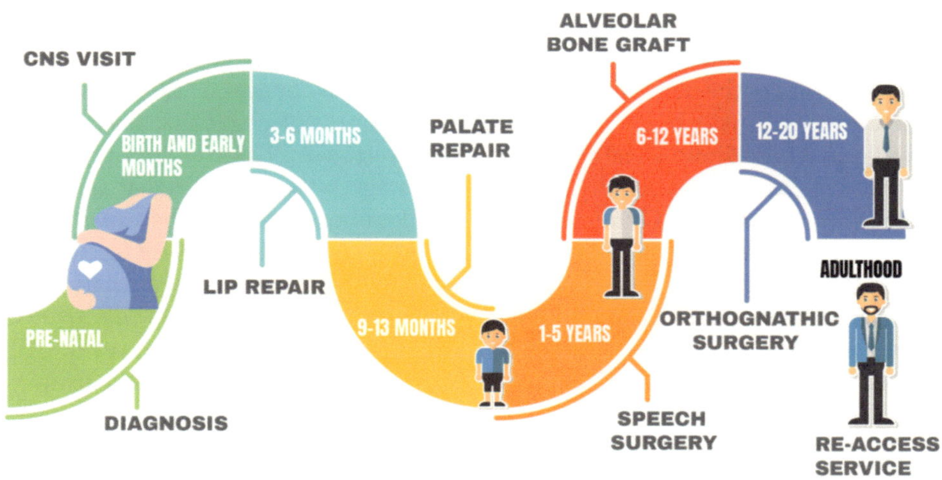

Figure 7.
A diagram simplifying the cleft pathway in the United Kingdom.

is complete. After skeletal maturity, patients may have orthognathic surgery and other remedial operations. A multidisciplinary team provides care, which includes ongoing follow-up and support [67].

6.1 Preoperative management

Breastfeeding is recommended for newborns with cleft palate, despite potential feeding difficulties and a higher risk of aspiration, and mothers should seek assistance from qualified lactation consultants [68]. Specialised bottles and teats can help with feeding, and carers should advise infants to eat in an upright position to avoid the risk of reflux. Infants with orofacial clefts are expected to develop and gain weight similarly to their unaffected counterparts, while failure to thrive may postpone surgical intervention and increase the risk of postoperative complications [27, 69]. To aid in surgical preparation, cleft teams in some countries may offer NAM therapy, which uses the newborn's malleable oral tissues to realign nasal cartilage and align alveolar ridges, narrowing the cleft lip defect. NAM generally begins within the first week of life and lasts 3 to 6 months, with a custom-made acrylic plate changed every 2 weeks [37].

6.2 Goals of cleft palate repair

The primary goals of cleft palate repair remain consistent: to separate the oral and nasal cavities and reconstruct the velopharyngeal valve, thereby facilitating feeding, preventing malnutrition, and supporting speech development and social integration [70]. Despite differing views on surgical techniques, key principles are widely accepted: anatomical closure of the defect, tension-free suturing, reorientation of soft palate muscles to restore the levator veli palatini, lengthening and retro-positioning of the soft palate, minimising exposed bone and mucosa, and layered closure of both the hard and soft palate [70–73].

6.3 Surgical techniques

6.3.1 Single stage vs. two stage repair

The time and technique of cleft palate surgery are still being debated, with the focus on balancing the benefits of early speech development against the risk of delayed maxillary growth. Early palatal repair improves speech results, although delayed repair may diminish iatrogenic midfacial retrusion. There are two primary techniques to palatoplasty: single-stage and two-stage, with strategies that are customised to the severity and kind of cleft. Schweckendiek developed the two-stage repair between 1944 and 1951, which consists of early soft palate closure (generally between 5 and 17 months) to promote speech, followed by delayed hard palate repair (typically between 18 and 36 months) to protect facial growth. Ross [74] discovered near-normal dental arches in Schweckendiek's patients, although Bardach et al. [75] reported major speech difficulties, possibly related to very late hard palate closure (about 16 years). Variations of this strategy are still used today [76–80].

Some centres in the United Kingdom and the Oslo Cleft Palate Team, use a modified two-stage protocol: early lip repair with a single-layer hard palate closure using a vomer flap at 3 months, followed by soft palate repair at 18 months [81, 82], with the goal of minimising growth restriction [83–88]. The single-stage method, sometimes known as "hole-in-one" repair, includes simultaneously closing the hard and soft palates at roughly 10 months of age. This approach is extensively used, particularly in resource-constrained environments where multiple procedures are difficult [89, 90]. Around 88–96% of cleft surgeons in the United States perform single-stage palatoplasty, with the average age of surgery being around 10 months [76].

Evidence suggests similar rates of orthognathic surgery following single- and two-stage approaches (20.8 vs. 21%), but VPI and need for speech surgery are higher after two-stage repairs (23.9 vs. 15.1%) [91]. Numerous studies have confirmed that early repair leads to better speech outcomes, though concerns about midfacial retrusion remain. Despite extensive research, there is no universally accepted protocol for palatoplasty. Surgical techniques vary widely across centres and are often modified or combined according to individual surgeon preference and patient needs [92]. The next sections will outline current international practices and propose a simplified algorithm to clarify the range of approaches to cleft palate repair.

6.3.2 Von Langenbeck palatoplasty

Bernard von Langenbeck proposed a palatoplasty technique that utilised mucoperiosteal flaps in 1861 (**Figure 8**). Incisions are made along the medial cleft edges, followed by lateral relaxing incisions to elevate the mucoperiosteum, resulting in bipedicled flaps for mouth closure. Muscle restoration is accomplished with intravelar veloplasty, and the nasal mucosa is mobilised for nasal closure. This approach is more

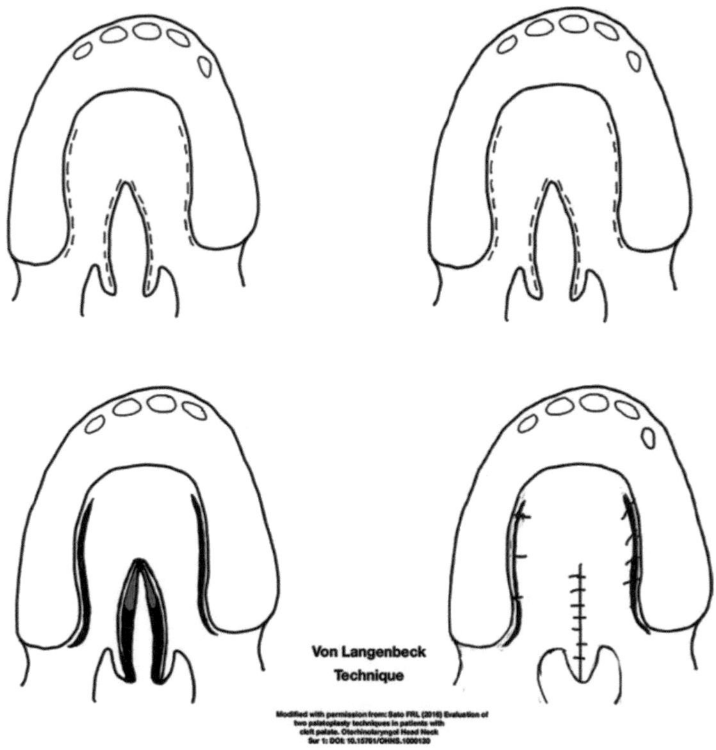

Figure 8.
Von Langenbeck's palatoplasty technique (drawn by the first author, modified from Ref. [93]).

appropriate for secondary palate clefts because bipedicled flaps are insufficient for primary palate closure [92, 94–97].

Advantages:

- Simple, well-established technique.
- Effective in secondary palatal clefts.
- Allows for muscle repair via intravelar veloplasty.
- Reliable bipedicled flap design.

Disadvantages:

- Limited tissue mobilisation makes it unsuitable for primary clefts.
- Less effective for large clefts due to restricted reach.
- May not provide adequate length for velopharyngeal competence.

6.3.3 Bardach two-flap palatoplasty

This procedure, a variation on the Von Langenbeck palatoplasty (**Figure 9**), includes deploying the entire hard palate as bilateral monopedicled mucoperiosteal flaps that are closed along the midline and vascularised by the larger palatine arteries [73]. It is appropriate for complete unilateral and bilateral clefts, allowing for two-layer closure and fistula repair at the posterior alveolus. The levator veli palatini muscle is dissected and repaired to re-establish the muscular sling using intravelar veloplasty principles [98]. One significant advantage is its ability to cover both primary and secondary palatal clefts; yet, it may be prone to problems due to varying flap vascularity. While it is frequently used for hard palate repair, it may be less effective than the Furlow approach for soft palate lengthening. It can also be coupled with vomer flaps to close the nasal mucosa [72, 98].

Advantages:

- Suitable for complete unilateral and bilateral clefts.
- Allows two-layer closure with better tension-free healing.
- Effective for both primary and secondary cleft repairs.
- Provides good access for levator muscle reconstruction.

Disadvantages:

- Flap vascularity may be variable, increasing risk of complications.
- Less effective in soft palate lengthening compared to Furlow technique.
- Potential for flap compromise in extensive clefts.

DOI: http://dx.doi.org/10.5772/intechopen.1012388

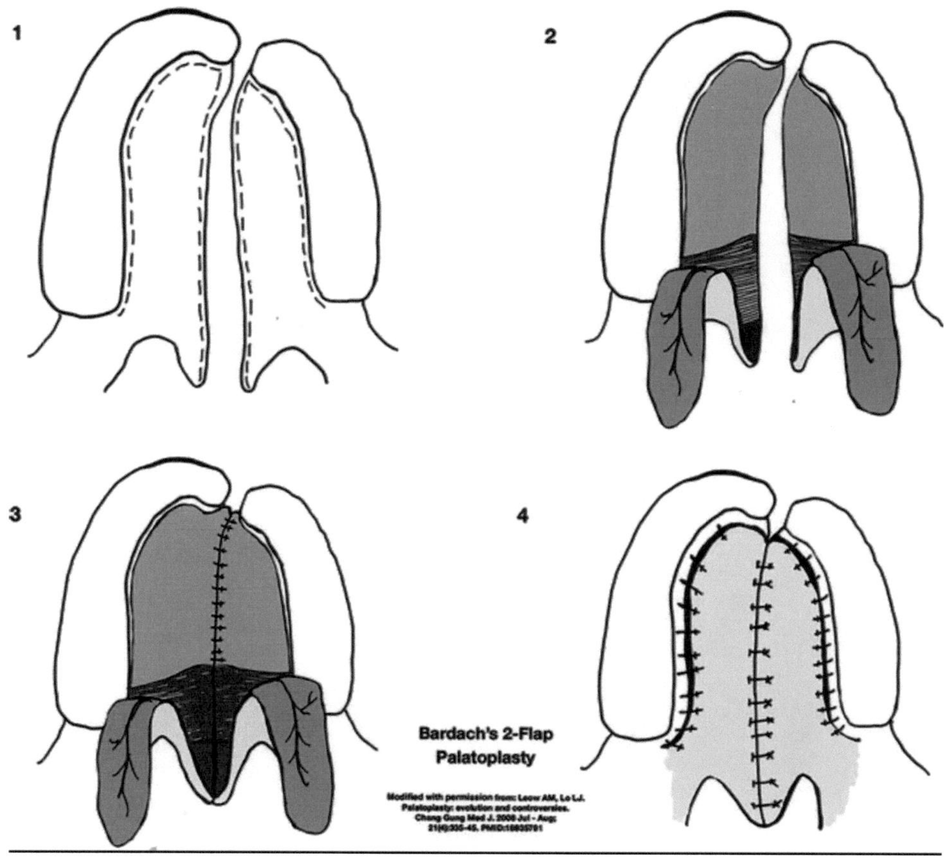

Figure 9.
Bardach's two-flap palatoplasty technique (drawn by the first author, modified from Ref. [77]).

6.3.4 Veau–Wardill–Kilner Palatoplasty (V to Y pushback)

The Veau–Wardill–Kilner approach is a variation of the von Langenbeck method that includes a V–Y pushback closure of the anterior hard palate (**Figure 10**). It converts bipedicled flaps to unipedicled ones by releasing the anterior palate at the intersection of the primary and secondary palates [99]. While this method allows for more advancement and extension of the palate, it leaves a significant raw region anteriorly and laterally along the alveolar margin, exposing the underlying membranous bone. This region heals with secondary intention, which might result in palatal shortening and velopharyngeal incompetence. Furthermore, the bare surface next to the alveolar ridge may cause alveolar arch abnormalities and dental misalignment [98].

Advantages:

- Achieves significant palatal lengthening.
- Converts bipedicled to unipedicled flaps for enhanced mobility.
- Useful in wide clefts requiring more posterior reach.

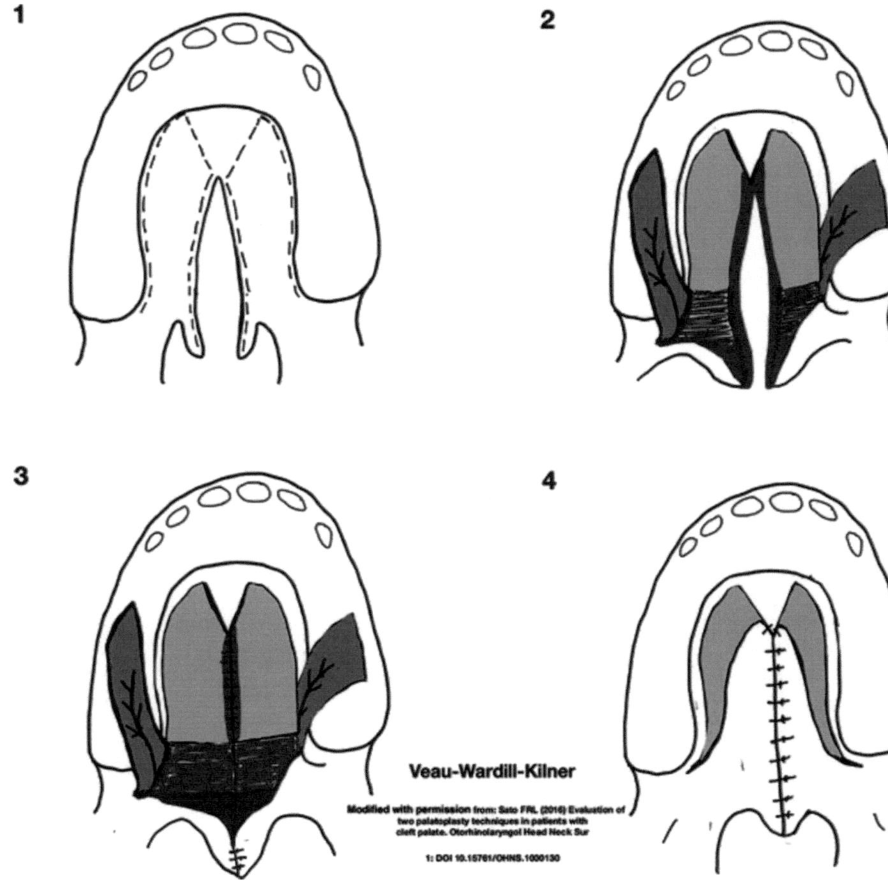

Figure 10.
Veau–Wardill–Kilner palatoplasty technique (drawn by the first author, modified from Ref. [93]).

Disadvantages:

- Leaves raw areas anteriorly and laterally that heal by secondary intention.
- May lead to velopharyngeal incompetence due to scar contracture.
- Associated with dental arch disturbances and malalignment.

6.3.5 Furlow double-opposing Z-plasty

The Furlow approach is a technically rigorous treatment that uses a double-opposing Z-plasty to lengthen the soft palate, making it especially successful for treating isolated clefts of the secondary soft palate and secondary repair of VPI (**Figure 11**) [70, 100]. The treatment involves making mirror-image Z-plasty incisions on both the oral and nasal surfaces, which allows the levator veli palatini muscles to be repositioned from sagittal to transverse orientations. This reconfiguration not only lengthens the palate but also helps to restore normal muscle function. One prominent result of this method is a reduction in the intertonsillar distance, which may diminish the palate's transverse breadth. The Furlow approach consistently improves soft palate length and velopharyngeal function, but it can cause tension when used to heal large

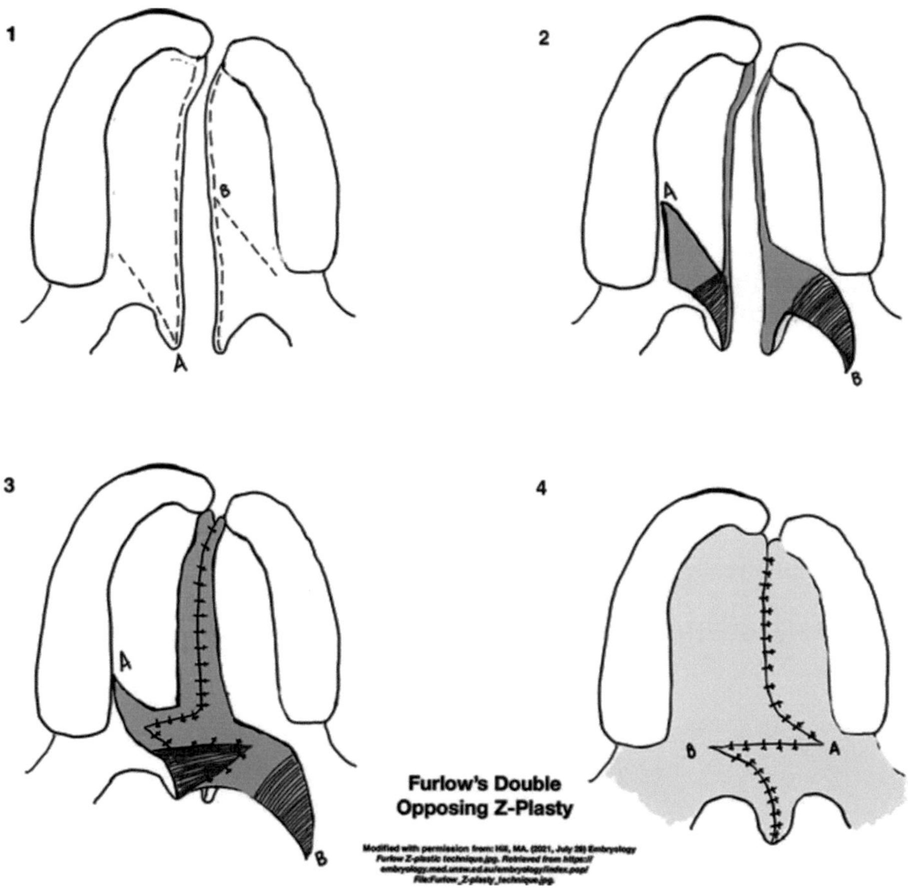

Figure 11.
Furlow's double-opposing Z-plasty technique (drawn by the first author, modified from Hill MA et al.).

clefts. While it can be paired with other methods, such as Bardach's, it is not optimal for large bilateral clefts and requires careful patient selection [88].

Advantages:

- Provides excellent soft palate lengthening.
- Anatomically repositions the levator muscle for improved speech outcomes.
- Ideal for isolated soft palate clefts and VPI repair.
- Minimises risk of midline scar contracture.

Disadvantages:

- Technically demanding with longer operative time.
- Less suitable for large or bilateral clefts due to tension.
- May reduce transverse width of the palate (intertonsillar narrowing).

6.3.6 Intravelar veloplasty

In 1968, Braithwaite described dissecting the levator veli palatini muscle from the posterior margin of the hard palate and surrounding mucosa, placing it posteriorly, and suturing it independently to restore the levator sling [101]. This method, known as intravelar veloplasty, has since been developed by many surgeons seeking more exact anatomical repair (**Figure 12**). Notably, Sommerlad advises for a major microscopic incision of the levator muscle belly with separate suturing, emphasising its critical role in elevating the soft palate during speaking. Intravelar veloplasty is considered a technical refinement in muscle reconstruction rather than a unique surgery. While it improves soft palate function and may help with VPI, the resulting midline scar may limit palatal movement [103].

Advantages:

- Allows precise anatomical levator muscle restoration.
- Enhances soft palate elevation and velopharyngeal function.
- Can be integrated into multiple palatoplasty techniques.
- Microsurgical refinements improve outcomes.

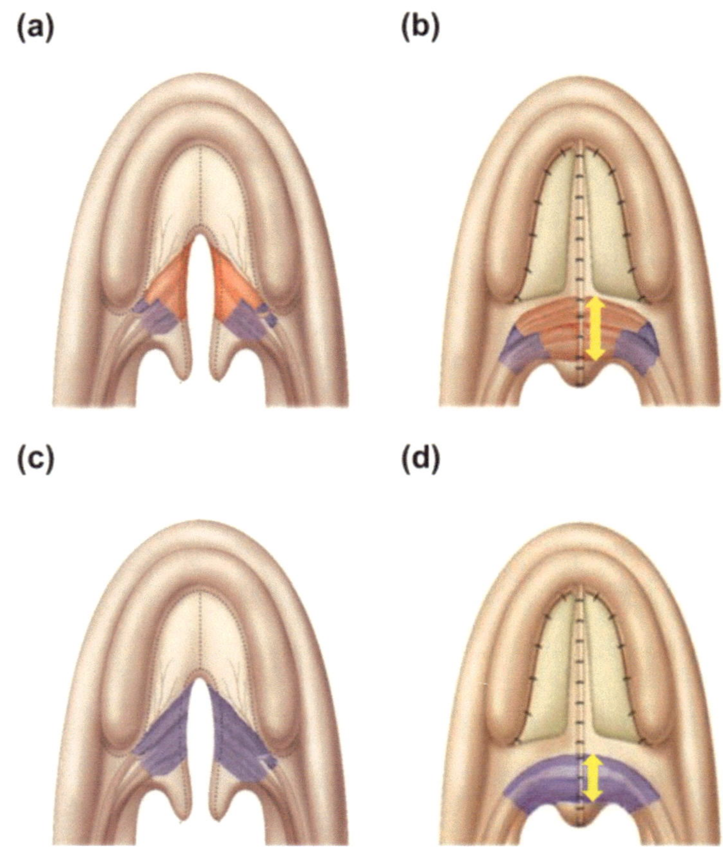

Figure 12.
Intravelar veloplasty technique (drawn by the first author, modified from Hill MA et al. Ref. [102]).

Disadvantages:

- Adds technical complexity.
- Midline scarring may still impair palatal motion.
- Not a standalone technique—requires integration with flap repair.

6.3.7 Vomer flap

The vomerine mucoperiosteal tissue is extremely versatile (**Figure 13**). Most surgeons utilise the vomer flap to close clefts in the anterior hard palate and alveolar areas. In these regions, the vomer flap is commonly used as a superior turnover flap. Recently, there has been renewed interest in this tissue, and its use has expanded to include more palatal abnormalities. Several forms of vomer flaps have been described for use in both unilateral and bilateral cleft palates, with applications, including nasal lining repair and oral mucosa resurfacing [70].

Advantages:

- Versatile flap for anterior hard palate and nasal lining closure.
- Useful in both unilateral and bilateral clefts.
- Reduces oronasal fistula rate.
- Expands reconstructive options with various orientations.

Disadvantages:

- Limited to areas where vomer tissue is adequate.
- May require combination with other flaps for full closure.
- Risk of overuse inappropriately replacing more robust nasal repairs.

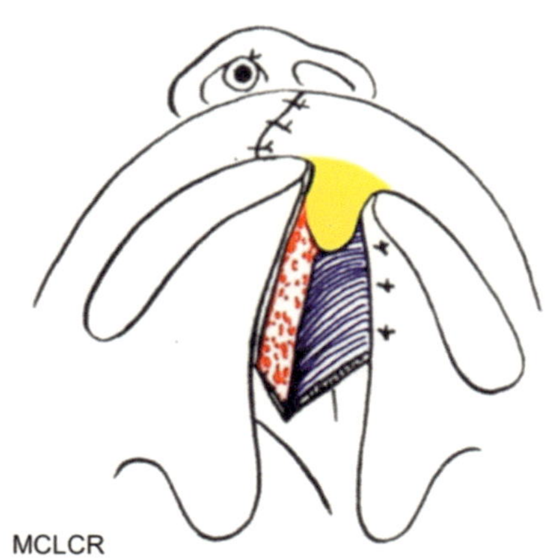

Figure 13.
A diagram showing the turnover septal flap (vomer flap) in blue. The stripped red area is the raw area on the septum. Ref. [104] under Creative Commons Attribution-NonCommercial-ShareAlike 3.0 Unported Licence (CC BY-NC-SA 3.0).

6.4 Postoperative plan

The majority of patients are hospitalised overnight for observation after cleft palate surgery. A soft diet is recommended for 1 month after surgery, and straws should be avoided to protect the surgical site from irritation and infection. The timing of postoperative evaluations varies according to the individual patient's health, as well as the surgeon's training and prior experience with similar situations. Most patients are reassessed 2 weeks after surgery [105].

6.5 Complications

6.5.1 Immediate (within 2 weeks of surgical repair)

- Postoperative airway obstruction following cleft palate repair might be caused by tongue or palatal oedema. In the supine posture, a large tongue might fall back and impede the airway. Prolonged intubation and postoperative ventilation may be required, especially in syndromic patients with comorbidities or intraoperative instability, necessitating care in a paediatrics ICU [106].

- Laryngospasm, a known concern after upper aerodigestive procedures, can occur during extubating and usually responds to positive-pressure ventilation. Reintubation may also be necessary.

- Gentle pressure is often used to treat haemorrhage, which occurs when blood pressure rises and dislodges clots from the palate.

- Excessive stress or trauma might cause wound dehiscence during the repair process.

- Infection can cause fistulas or visible symptoms like redness, warmth, purulent discharge, and pain [107].

6.5.2 Long-term ($\geq$ 2 weeks after surgical repair)

- Palatal fistulas are aberrant connections between the oral and nasal cavities caused by local repair failure, infection, or trauma following palate surgery. The Pittsburgh Fistula Classification System distinguishes seven anatomical categories of fistulae, from the uvula (Type I) to the labial-alveolar area (Type VII). This system is anatomical in nature and does not account for symptoms. The treatment depends on whether the fistula is symptomatic. Asymptomatic fistulae seldom require therapy, whereas symptomatic ones frequently necessitate surgical correction; however, recurrence is typical even in minor defects [108].

- Inadequate palatal mobility after surgery can prevent the velopharyngeal port from closing properly during speaking. This could be due to inadequate tissue handling, extensive scarring, insufficient healing, or underlying neurological problems. Finally, palatal necrosis is an uncommon but serious complication caused by damage to the larger palatine artery during the flap elevation procedure. Necrosis can occur immediately or after a delay, with fatal consequences [107].

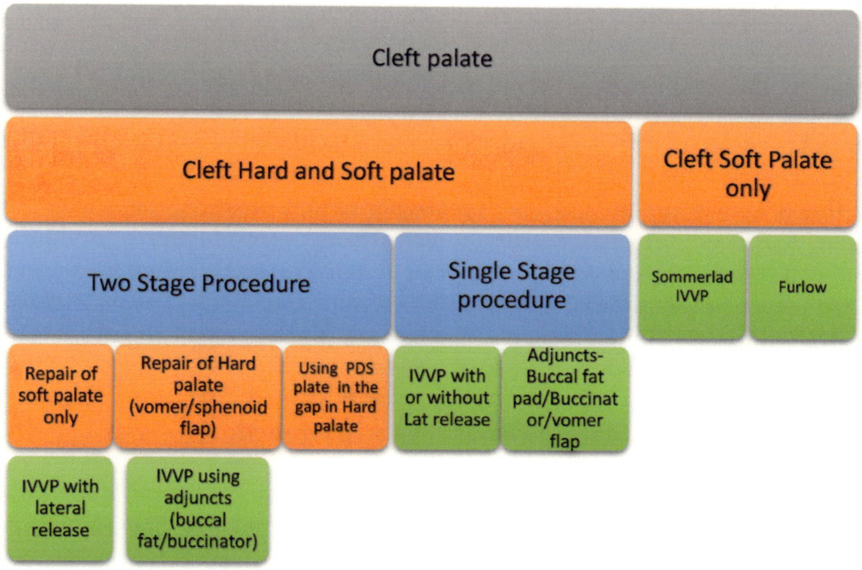

Figure 14.
Algorithm for the surgical management of different types of cleft palate considering the most common techniques worldwide.

6.6 Long-term outcomes

Timbang et al. conducted a comprehensive review that compared the long-term outcomes of cleft palate repair using the Furlow double-opposing Z-plasty and straight-line intravelar veloplasty. From an initial 5911 studies, 12 fulfilled the inclusion requirements, including 927 Furlow and 1205 straight-line repairs. The Furlow group had a slightly lower overall oronasal fistula rate (7.87%) than the straight-line group (9.81%), but the difference was not statistically significant ($p = 0.14$). Speech outcomes, measured primarily by the need for secondary VPI surgery and the presence of hypernasality, favoured the Furlow method, with lower secondary surgery rates (0–11.4% vs. 6.7–29.2%) and less hypernasality, especially in unilateral cleft lip-palate patients, where the difference in secondary surgery rates reached statistical significance ($p = 0.03$). Despite differences across trials, Furlow repair generally resulted in superior functional outcomes [108].

6.7 Palatal repair algorithm

Developing an algorithm for palate repair is particularly challenging due to the wide range of surgical techniques available and the lack of consensus regarding the effectiveness of each method for repairing both the soft and hard palate. This is, therefore, a modest attempt to simplify and illustrate the various techniques, rather than to provide a precise or definitive description (**Figure 14**).

7. Velopharyngeal dysfunction

Velopharyngeal dysfunction (VPD) occurs when the dynamic structures responsible for controlling the velopharyngeal (VP) sphincter, which include the soft palate, lateral pharyngeal walls, and posterior pharyngeal wall, fail to function properly, preventing proper separation of the nasal and oral cavities during speech. The levator veli palatini, tensor veli palatini, palatoglossus, palatopharyngeus, musculus uvulae, salpingopharyngeus, and superior pharyngeal constrictors all have a role in VP sphincter function [109]. These muscles work together to regulate air pressure and sound generated by the respiratory system, shaping and directing airflow and resonance between the oral and nasal canals to produce understandable speech. When this system is impaired, it can cause hypernasal resonance, abnormal nasal air emission, decreased intraoral pressure, which affects the production of oral pressure consonants, reduced speech loudness, nostril or facial grimacing, hyperfunctional changes to voice production, or the development of maladaptive speech patterns [110]. Approximately 30% of patients who have cleft palate repair require secondary surgery for VPD, with VPI being the most prevalent variant [88, 111].

7.1 Diagnosis and evaluation of velopharyngeal dysfunction

A multidisciplinary team should address VPD by using a variety of diagnostic methods to assess speech outcomes both before and after surgery. Speech pathologists play an important role in identifying the difference between speech irregularities caused by structural disorders that may benefit from surgery and those that require behavioural therapy. A speech-language pathologist (SLP) will do an initial examination that includes perceptual speech analysis, with an emphasis on pressure sounds, nasal consonants, and resonance patterns. Misarticulations are examined for developmental, compensatory, or anatomical causes, and aberrant nasal emissions or facial grimacing are identified [112]. Objective tests such as nasometry give repeatable data on nasal emissions by comparing nasal and oral sound emissions before and after surgery, but they do not identify the source or location of the VP gap [113].

Advanced imaging techniques aid in the diagnosis of VPD. Video nasopharyngeal endoscopy (VNPE) provides direct, high-quality visualisation of VP structures during speech, such as closure patterns and muscle activity [114–116]. Multiview speech videofluoroscopy (MVSVF) enhances VNPE by giving two-dimensional imaging of the VP sphincter, as well as additional information about velar motion, adenoid size, and pharyngeal wall movement, especially when contrast is employed [117]. Magnetic resonance imaging (MRI) provides radiation-free, comprehensive anatomical insights on VP structures such as levator muscle orientation and pharyngeal depth. However, its dynamic image quality may not be as good as videofluoroscopy, and its high cost and scarcity limit its utilisation. These methodologies work together to provide a comprehensive assessment and provide individualised management recommendations for patients with VPD [118–121].

7.2 Treatment of velopharyngeal dysfunction (VPD)

The management of VPD is customised to the underlying cause, with the goal of improving speech outcomes [122, 123]. Speech therapy, prosthetic devices, surgery, or a mix of the three, are all viable treatment options. A thorough diagnostic examination is required to determine the most appropriate therapy [117].

7.2.1 Nonsurgical management

Patients who are not candidates for surgery can benefit from prosthetic devices, which provide temporary or permanent treatments. These bespoke devices might function as palatal lifts, obturators, or speech bulbs. Palatal lifts help to elevate the soft palate, which is effective in cases of hypomobility or paralysis, whereas obturators close oronasal fistulae or unrepaired cleft. When more surgery is not an option, speech bulbs can help to close chronic abnormalities. Speech therapy is still necessary, particularly for treating VP mislearning, and it is frequently required postoperatively to assist patients to adapt to their repaired anatomy and resolve maladaptive articulation [117].

7.2.2 Surgical management

Surgical therapy aims to address either a short palate or decreased palatal mobility. This usually entails lengthening the palate with techniques like buccal myomucosal flaps or Furlow palatoplasty, or augmenting the posterior pharyngeal wall with procedures like a posterior pharyngeal flap, sphincter pharyngoplasty, or fat grafting.

7.2.2.1 Buccal myomucosal flaps (BMMFs)

The buccinator myomucosal flap (BMMF) (**Figure 15**) is a pedicled, intraoral flap that is increasingly being employed in palatal lengthening to treat VPI after palatoplasty, particularly in patients with an intact but poorly positioned levator sling or insufficient velar length. The surgery entails disjunction of the hard-soft palate junction, followed by elevation of bilateral BMMFs from the inner cheek. These flaps are created by making parallel incisions 5–7 mm above and below the level of the parotid duct, stretching from the retromolar trigone anteriorly towards the oral commissure, and then elevating in a submucosal plane to incorporate buccinator muscle fibres. The flap's posterior base is carefully preserved to provide venous supply. Once elevated, the flaps are turned medially and posteriorly to enhance the soft palate's nasal surface, allowing for posterior levator sling repositioning and efficient velar lengthening. This approach has various advantages, including the use of vascularised, unscarred tissue, little donor site morbidity, a lower risk of scar contracture due to the small raw area, and the retention of the nasopharyngeal port. Furthermore, it is reversible and can be lengthened as needed. Jackson et al. described the successful use of a unilateral BMMF during primary palatoplasty with excellent speech outcomes and minimal fistula rates, emphasising its adaptability not just as a salvage operation but also as a primary adjunct [122, 123, 125–128].

7.2.2.2 Furlow double-opposing Z-plasty

This method realigns and rebuilds the levator muscle sling to restore function. Elevating and reorienting mucosal and muscular flaps repositions the levator muscle transversely, overlapping over the midline, hence improving VP closure [117].

7.2.2.3 Posterior pharyngeal flap (PPF)

Previously, the first-line surgical treatment for VPI, the PPF is currently only used for individuals who have palatal paralysis or residual VPI after BMMF surgery. The PPF provides a soft tissue bridge between the posterior pharynx and soft palate, resulting in two smaller lateral ports that restrict airflow during speaking. Success is

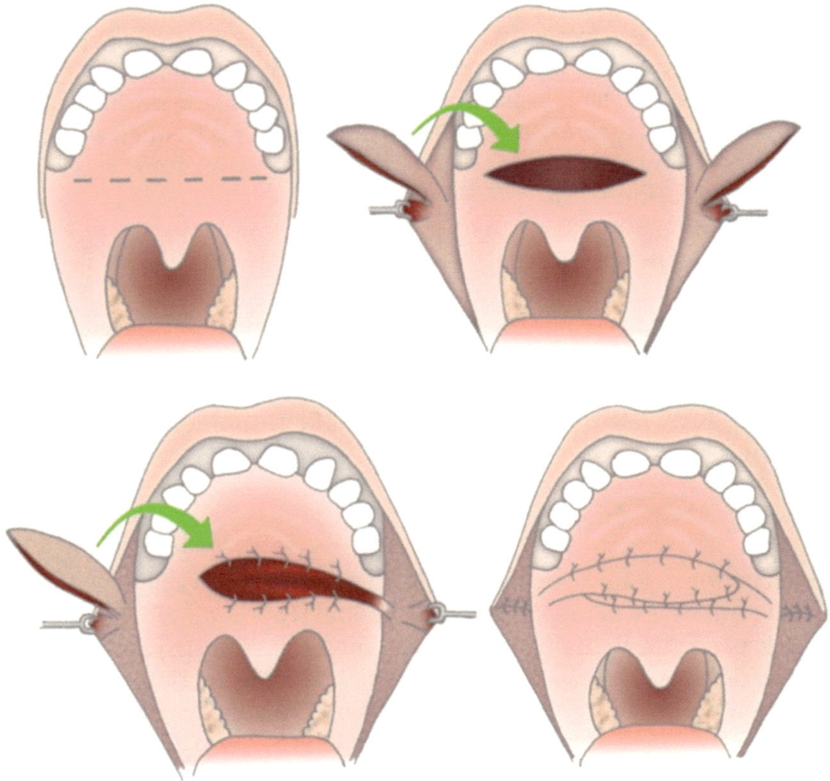

Figure 15.
Steps of raising bilateral buccal myomucosal flap. Ref. [124].

dependent on adequate lateral pharyngeal wall mobility [129–131]. A superiorly based flap is favoured for increased surgical exposure and a longer flap harvest [132, 133].

7.2.2.4 Sphincter pharyngoplasty

This method is utilised on individuals who have tiny VP gaps and limited lateral pharyngeal wall mobility. Vertically orientated posterior tonsillar pillar flaps (palatopharyngeus muscles) are twisted medially to generate a dynamic sphincter, which is occasionally supplemented with the longus capitis muscle and polypropylene cerclage sutures. While it efficiently narrows the velopharyngeal port, there is a risk of increased scarring and irreversible airway narrowing [134–137].

7.2.2.5 Augmentation of the posterior pharyngeal wall and soft palate

Autologous tissue grafts, such as fat, cartilage, and dermis, are now preferred over synthetic materials because to their lower extrusion rates. However, there is limited data to support their long-term efficacy. This approach is most suited for patients who have modest VP gaps [138–141].

In conclusion, the surgical correction of VPD demands an individualised approach based on anatomical and neurological factors, VP gap size, closure pattern, levator sling status, and the surgeon's expertise.

8. Conclusion

The management of cleft palate is inherently multidisciplinary, requiring the coordinated efforts of a wide range of healthcare professionals, such as surgeons, speech and language therapists, orthodontists, audiologists, and paediatricians. Given the complexity and long-term nature of treatment, which often spans from infancy through adolescence, it is inevitable that any medical professional involved in the care of paediatric patients will, at some stage, play a role in the management or support of a child with a cleft condition. Whether directly involved in surgical intervention or in providing ongoing support and monitoring, healthcare providers across specialties must be familiar with the needs and challenges faced by this patient group to ensure comprehensive, holistic care.

Conflict of interest

The authors declare no conflict of interest.

Author details

Samar Mousa[1*] and Nitisha Narayan[2]

1 Specialty Trainee in Plastic Surgery, North Bristol NHS Trust, Southwest Deanery, United Kingdom

2 Consultant Cleft, Plastic and Reconstructive Surgeon, Southwest Cleft Service, Bristol, UK

*Address all correspondence to: samar.mousa@nhs.net

References

[1] Kenhub. The Soft Palate: Anatomy, Function and Clinical Aspects [Internet]. Kenhub. Available from: https://www.kenhub.com/en/library/anatomy/the-soft-palate [Accessed: June 29, 2025]

[2] Phalke N, Goldman JJ. Cleft palate. In: StatPearls [Internet]. Treasure Island (FL): StatPearls Publishing; 2024. p. 2025

[3] Gray H. The development of the face. In: Gray's Anatomy. [Internet]. Wikimedia Commons; 2006 [Accessed: May 6, 2025]. Available from: https://commons.wikimedia.org/wiki/File:Gray1201.png

[4] Gray H. The roof of the mouth. In: Gray's Anatomy. [Internet]. Wikimedia Commons; 2006. Available from: https://commons.wikimedia.org/wiki/File:Gray160.png [Accessed: May 6, 2025]

[5] Veau V. Division Palatine: Anatomie, Chirurgie, Phonétique. Paris: Masson; 1931

[6] Kernahan DA, Stark RB. A new classification for cleft lip and cleft palate. Plastic and Reconstructive Surgery and the Transplantation Bulletin. 1958;**22**:435-441

[7] Harkins CS, Berlin A, Harding RL, Longacre JJ, Snodgrasse RM. A classification of cleft lip and cleft palate. Plastic and Reconstructive Surgery and the Transplantation Bulletin. 1962;**29**:31-39. DOI: 10.1097/00006534-196201000-00005

[8] Helwany M, Rathee M. Anatomy, head and neck, palate. In: StatPearls [Internet]. Treasure Island (FL): StatPearls Publishing; 2025. Available from: https://www.ncbi.nlm.nih.gov/books/NBK557817/ [Accessed: June 5, 2023]

[9] Gray H. The arteries of the back of the forearm. In: Gray's Anatomy. Philadelphia: Lea & Febiger; 1918. Available from: https://commons.wikimedia.org/wiki/File:Gray1028.png

[10] Cho JH, Kim JK, Lee HY, Yoon JH. Surgical anatomy of human soft palate. The Laryngoscope. 2013;**123**(11):2900-2904. DOI: 10.1002/lary.24067. Epub 2013 May 17

[11] Shigeta Y, Ogawa T, Tomoko I, Clark GT, Enciso R. Soft palate length and upper airway relationship in OSA and non-OSA subjects. Sleep & Breathing. 2010;**14**(4):353-358. DOI: 10.1007/s11325-009-0318-7. Epub 2009 Dec 8

[12] Mercer NS, MacCarthy P. The arterial supply of the palate: Implications for closure of cleft palates. Plastic and Reconstructive Surgery. 1995;**96**(5):1038-1044. DOI: 10.1097/00006534-199510000-00005

[13] Zhong W, Zhang K, Wang F. Applied anatomical study of blood supply in human palate. Zhonghua Kou Qiang Yi Xue Za Zhi. 2001;**36**(2):136-138. Chinese

[14] Mu L, Chen J, Li J, Arnold M, Sobotka S, Nyirenda T, et al. Sensory innervation of the human soft palate. Anatomical Record (Hoboken, N.J.: 2007). 2018;**301**(11):1861-1870. DOI: 10.1002/ar.23864. Epub 2018 Aug 6

[15] Craniofacial Team of Texas. Embryology: Palate Formation. Craniofacial Team of Texas. [Internet]; [Accessed: May 6, 2025]. Available from: https://craniofacialteamtexas.com/cleft-lip-and-cleft-palate/

what-causes-cleft-lips-and-palates/embryology-palate-formation/

[16] Dursun A, Öztürk K, Albay S. Development of hard and soft palate during the fetal period and hard palate asymmetry. The Journal of Craniofacial Surgery. 2018;**29**(8):2358-2362. DOI: 10.1097/SCS.0000000000005016

[17] Greene RM, Pisano MM. Palate morphogenesis: Current understanding and future directions. Birth Defects Research. Part C, Embryo Today. 2010;**90**(2):133-154. DOI: 10.1002/bdrc.20180

[18] Matsumoto R, Evans SE. The palatal dentition of tetrapods and its functional significance. Journal of Anatomy. 2017;**230**(1):47-65. DOI: 10.1111/joa.12534. Epub 2016 Aug 19

[19] Hammond NL, Dixon MJ. Revisiting the embryogenesis of lip and palate development. Oral Diseases. 2022;**28**(5):1306-1326. DOI: 10.1111/odi.14174. Epub 2022 Mar 5

[20] Kirschner RE, LaRossa D. Cleft lip and palate. Otolaryngologic Clinics of North America. 2000;**33**(6):1191-1215, v-vi. DOI: 10.1016/s0030-6665(05)70277-2

[21] Gritli-Linde A. Molecular control of secondary palate development. Developmental Biology. 2007;**301**(2):309-326. DOI: 10.1016/j.ydbio.2006.07.042. Epub 2006 Aug 5

[22] Zhang Z, Stein M, Mercer N, Malic C. Post-operative outcomes after cleft palate repair in syndromic and non-syndromic children: A systematic review protocol. Systematic Reviews. 2017;**6**(1):52. DOI: 10.1186/s13643-017-0438-2

[23] Centers for Disease Control and Prevention. Orofacial clefts: Cleft palate. In: Birth Defects Surveillance Manual: Quick Reference Handbook. Atlanta (GA): CDC; 2022. Available from: https://archive.cdc.gov/www_cdc_gov/ncbddd/birthdefects/surveillancemanual/quick-reference-handbook/cleft-palate.html

[24] Applebaum SA, Aronson S, Termanini KM, Gosain AK. Evidence-based practices in cleft palate surgery. Plastic and Reconstructive Surgery. 2024;**153**(2):448e-461e. DOI: 10.1097/PRS.0000000000011035. Epub 2024 Jan 24

[25] Vanlam FS, Bendeus M, Wong RW. A multidisciplinary team approach on cleft lip and palate management. Hong Kong Dental Journal. 2007;**4**(1):38-45

[26] Mahboubi H, Truong A, Pham NS. Prevalence, demographics, and complications of cleft palate surgery. International Journal of Pediatric Otorhinolaryngology. 2015;**79**(6):803-807. DOI: 10.1016/j.ijporl.2015.02.032. Epub 2015 Mar 6

[27] Lewis CW, Jacob LS, Lehmann CU, Section on Oral Health. The primary care pediatrician and the care of children with cleft lip and/or cleft palate. Pediatrics. 2017;**139**(5):e20170628. DOI: 10.1542/peds.2017-0628. Erratum in: Pediatrics. 2017 Sep;140(3):e20171921. DOI: 10.1542/peds.2017-1921

[28] Shkoukani MA, Chen M, Vong A. Cleft lip - A comprehensive review. Frontiers in Pediatrics. 2013;**1**:53. DOI: 10.3389/fped.2013.00053

[29] World Health Organization. International Collaborative Research on Craniofacial Anomalies. Available from: www.who.int/genomics/anomalies/en [Accessed: May 2, 2025]

[30] Salari N, Darvishi N, Heydari M, Bokaee S, Darvishi F, Mohammadi M. Global prevalence of cleft palate, cleft lip and cleft palate and lip: A comprehensive

systematic review and meta-analysis. Journal of Stomatology, Oral and Maxillofacial Surgery. 2022;**123**(2):110-120. DOI: 10.1016/j.jormas.2021.05.008. Epub 2021 May 24

[31] Cleft Registry and Audit NEtwork (CRANE). CRANE Database 2024 Annual Report [Internet]. London: Clinical Effectiveness Unit, Royal College of Surgeons of England; 2024. Available from: https://www.crane-database.org.uk/reports/crane-database-2024-annual-report/ [Accessed: May 2, 2025]

[32] Cleft Registry and Audit NEtwork (CRANE). CRANE Database 2020 Annual Report [Internet]. London: Clinical Effectiveness Unit, Royal College of Surgeons of England; 2020. Available from: https://www.crane-database.org.uk/reports/crane-database-2020-annual-report/ [Accessed: May 2, 2025]

[33] Woo AS. Evidence-based medicine: Cleft palate. Plastic and Reconstructive Surgery. 2017;**139**(1):191e-203e. DOI: 10.1097/PRS.0000000000002854

[34] Deshpande AS, Goudy SL. Cellular and molecular mechanisms of cleft palate development. Laryngoscope Investigative Otolaryngology. 2018;**4**(1):160-164. DOI: 10.1002/lio2.214

[35] Somerville N, Fenlon S. Anaesthesia for cleft lip and palate surgery. Pain. 2005;**5**:76-79

[36] Davis JS, Ritchie HP. Classification of congenital clefts of the lip and palate: With a suggestion for recording these cases. Journal of the American Medical Association. 1922;**79**(16):1323-1327. DOI: 10.1001/jama.1922.02640160043014

[37] Alois CI, Ruotolo RA. An overview of cleft lip and palate. JAAPA : Official Journal of the American Academy of Physician Assistants. 2020;**33**(12):17-20. DOI: 10.1097/01.JAA.0000721644.06681.06

[38] Allori AC, Mulliken JB, Meara JG, Shusterman S, Marcus JR. Classification of cleft lip/palate: Then and now. The Cleft Palate-Craniofacial Journal. 2017;**54**(2):175-188. DOI: 10.1597/14-080. Epub 2015 Sep 4

[39] Kernahan DA. The striped Y--A symbolic classification for cleft lip and palate. Plastic and Reconstructive Surgery. 1971;**47**(5):469-470. DOI: 10.1097/00006534-197105000-00010

[40] Elsahy NI. The modified striped Y—A systematic classification for cleft lip and palate. The Cleft Palate Journal. 1973;**10**:247-250

[41] Millard DR Jr. Cleft Craft: The Evolution of Its Surgery. Volume I: The Unilateral Deformity. Boston: Little, Brown and Company; 1976. ISBN: 0316571377

[42] Houkes RP, Hens G, Kubon C, Heliövaara A, Dávidovics K, Akota I, et al. Learnability of the LAHSHAL classification for oral clefts: Results of an international webinar. The Journal of Craniofacial Surgery. 2025;**36**(8):3032-3035. DOI: 10.1097/SCS.0000000000011355. Epub ahead of print

[43] World Health Organization. Global Health Estimates 2016: Disease Burden by Cause, Age, Sex, by Country and by Region, 2000-2016 [Internet]. Geneva: WHO; 2018. Available from: http://www.who.int/healthinfo/global_burden_disease/GHE2016_DALY_Global_2000_2016_.xls?ua=1 [Accessed: May 2, 2025]

[44] Truelsen T, Krarup LH, Iversen HK, Mensah GA, Feigin VL, Sposato LA, et al. Causes of death data in the

global burden of disease estimates for ischemic and hemorrhagic stroke. Neuroepidemiology. 2015;**45**(3):152-160. DOI: 10.1159/000441084. Epub 2015 Oct 28

[45] World Health Organization. International Statistical Classification of Diseases and Related Health Problems (ICD) [Internet]. Available from: https://www.who.int/standards/classifications/classification-of-diseases/ [Accessed: May 2, 2025]

[46] Houkes R, Smit J, Mossey P, Don Griot P, Persson M, Neville A, et al. Classification Systems of Cleft lip, alveolus and palate: Results of an international survey. The Cleft Palate-Craniofacial Journal. 2023;**60**(2):189-196. DOI: 10.1177/10556656211057368. Epub 2021 Nov 23

[47] Houkes R, Smit H, Mossey P, Don Griot P, Persson M, Neville A, et al. Classification systems of cleft lip, alveolus and palate: Results of an international survey. The Cleft Palate-Craniofacial Journal. 2021;**60**:105566562110573. DOI: 10.1177/10556656211057368

[48] American Speech-Language-Hearing Association. Comprehensive Assessment for Cleft Lip and Palate and Resonance [Internet]. Rockville (MD): ASHA; 2025. Available from: https://www.asha.org/practice-portal/resources/comprehensive-assessment-for-cleft-lip-and-palate-and-resonance/ [Accessed: May 2, 2025]

[49] McElroy H, Habel A, Jokinen M, Marsh C, Murphy G, Tuohy W. Improving the early detection of cleft palate in the UK [Internet]. Infant. 2017;**13**(6):223-227. Available from: https://www.infantjournal.co.uk/pdf/inf_078_tio.pdf [Accessed: May 2, 2025]

[50] Singh D, Bastian TS, Kudva S, Singh MK, Sharma P. Classification systems for orofacial clefts [Internet]. Oral and Maxillofacial Pathology Journal. 2015;**6**(1):556-560. Available from: https://www.ompj.org/files/c01b66a4126928dd63231a1ad32fadb4-6.pdf [Accessed: May 2, 2025]

[51] American Academy of Pediatric Dentistry. Policy on Management of Patients with Cleft Lip/Palate and Other Craniofacial Anomalies [Internet]. Chicago (IL): AAPD; 2018. Available from: https://www.aapd.org/media/policies_guidelines/e_cleftlip.pdf [Accessed: June 29, 2025]

[52] Kennelly MM, Moran P. Directional power Doppler in the midsagittal plane as an aid to the prenatal diagnosis of cleft lip and palate. Prenatal Diagnosis. 2008;**28**(1):56-58. DOI: 10.1002/pd.1892

[53] Johnson N, Sandy R, J. Prenatal diagnosis of cleft lip and palate. The Cleft Palate-Craniofacial Journal. 2003;**40**(2):186-189. DOI: 10.1597/1545-1569_2003_040_0186_pdocla_2.0.co_2

[54] Cash C, Set P, Coleman N. The accuracy of antenatal ultrasound in the detection of facial clefts in a low-risk screening population [Internet]. Ultrasound in Obstetrics & Gynecology. 2001;**18**(5):432-436. DOI: 10.1046/j.0960-7692.2001.00508.x [Accessed: May 2, 2025]

[55] Campbell S, Lees C, Moscoso G, Hall P. Ultrasound antenatal diagnosis of cleft palate by a new technique: The 3D 'reverse face' view. Ultrasound in Obstetrics & Gynecology. 2005;**25**(1):12-18. DOI: 10.1002/uog.1819

[56] Cleft Registry and Audit NEtwork. CRANE Database 2021 Annual Report. London: The Cleft Registry and Audit Network Clinical Effectiveness Unit (CEU), The Royal College of Surgeons of England; 2021. Available from: https://www.crane-database.org.uk/reports/crane-database-2021-annual-report/ [Accessed: May 2, 2025]

[57] Dudding T, Martin S, Popat S. An introduction to the UK care pathway for children born with a cleft of the lip and/or palate. British Dental Journal. 2023;**234**:943-946. DOI: 10.1038/s41415-023-5998-z

[58] Young JL, O'Riordan M, Goldstein JA, Robin NH. What information do parents of newborns with cleft lip, palate, or both want to know? The Cleft Palate-Craniofacial Journal. 2001;**38**(1):55-58. DOI: 10.1597/1545-1569_2001_038_0055_widpon_2.0.co_2

[59] Friede H, Johanson B. A follow-up study of cleft children treated with vomer flap as part of a three-stage soft tissue surgical procedure. Facial morphology and dental occlusion. Scandinavian Journal of Plastic and Reconstructive Surgery. 1977;**11**(1):45-57. DOI: 10.3109/02844317709025496

[60] Martin SV, Van Eeden S, Swan MC. The role of primary surgery in the management of orofacial clefting. British Dental Journal. 2023;**234**(12):859-866. DOI: 10.1038/s41415-023-6002-7. Epub 2023 Jun 23

[61] Haque S, Alam MK. Common dental anomalies in cleft lip and palate patients. The Malaysian Journal of Medical Sciences : MJMS. 2015;**22**(2):55-60

[62] Phippen G. Articulating the issues: Speech assessment and intervention in cleft lip and palate. British Dental Journal. 2023;**234**(12):912-917. DOI: 10.1038/s41415-023-5954-y. Epub 2023 Jun 23

[63] Wong Riff KWY, Tsangaris E, Forrest CR, Goodacre T, Longmire NM, Allen G, et al. CLEFT-Q: Detecting differences in outcomes among 2434 patients with varying cleft types. Plastic and Reconstructive Surgery. 2019;**144**(1):78e-88e. DOI: 10.1097/PRS.0000000000005723

[64] May J, Smallridge J, Collard M, Vaidyanathan M, Bhujel N. Challenges for dental care of the paediatric patient born with cleft lip and/or palate. British Dental Journal. 2023;**234**(12):867-871. DOI: 10.1038/s41415-023-5995-2. Epub 2023 Jun 23

[65] Popat S, Critchlow S. The restorative dentistry management of adult cleft patients: 'the adult returner'. British Dental Journal. 2023;**234**(12):906-911. DOI: 10.1038/s41415-023-5996-1. Epub 2023 Jun 23

[66] Schölin JS, Rizell S, Paganini A, Mark H. A national registry-based study of surgery and demography comparing internationally adopted and children born in Sweden with cleft lip and/or palate. Journal of Plastic Surgery and Hand Surgery. 2023;**57**(1-6):354-359. DOI: 10.1080/2000656X.2022.2097252

[67] Hattori Y, Pai BC, Saito T, Chou PY, Lu TC, Chang CS, et al. Long-term treatment outcome of patients with complete bilateral cleft lip and palate: A retrospective cohort study. International Journal of Surgery. 2023;**109**(6):1656-1667. DOI: 10.1097/JS9.0000000000000406

[68] Abbott BD. The etiology of cleft palate: A 50-year search for mechanistic and molecular understanding. Birth Defects Research. Part B, Developmental and Reproductive Toxicology. 2010;**89**(4):266-274. DOI: 10.1002/bdrb.20252

[69] Hammoudeh JA, Imahiyerobo TA, Liang F, Fahradyan A, Urbinelli L, Lau J, et al. Early cleft lip repair revisited: A safe and effective approach utilizing a multidisciplinary protocol. Plastic and Reconstructive Surgery. Global

Open. 2017;**5**(6):e1340. DOI: 10.1097/GOX.0000000000001340

[70] Agrawal K, Panda KN. Use of vomer flap in palatoplasty: Revisited. The Cleft Palate-Craniofacial Journal. 2006;**43**(1):30-37. DOI: 10.1597/04-034.1

[71] Tatum S, Senders C. Perspectives on palatoplasty. Facial Plastic Surgery. 1993;**9**(3):225-231. DOI: 10.1055/s-2008-1064617

[72] LaRossa D. The state of the art in cleft palate surgery. The Cleft Palate-Craniofacial Journal. 2000;**37**(3):225-228. DOI: 10.1597/1545-1569_2000_037_0225_tsotai_2.3.co_2

[73] Bardach J. Two-flap palatoplasty: Bardach's technique. Operative Techniques in Plastic and Reconstructive Surgery. 1995;**2**(4):211-214

[74] Ross RB. Treatment variables affecting facial growth in complete unilateral cleft lip and palate. The Cleft Palate Journal. 1987;**24**(1):5-77

[75] Bardach J, Bakowska J, McDermott-Murray J, Mooney MP, Dusdieker LB. Lip pressure changes following lip repair in infants with unilateral clefts of the lip and palate. Plastic and Reconstructive Surgery. 1984;**74**(4):476-481. DOI: 10.1097/00006534-198410000-00003

[76] Gundlach KKH, Bardach J, Filippow D, Stahl-de Castrillon F, Lenz JH. Two-stage palatoplasty, is it still a valuable treatment protocol for patients with a cleft of lip, alveolus, and palate? Journal of Cranio-Maxillo-Facial Surgery. 2013;**41**(1):62-70. DOI: 10.1016/j.jcms.2012.05.013

[77] Leow AM, Lo LJ. Palatoplasty: Evolution and controversies. Chang Gung Medical Journal. 2008;**31**(4):335-345

[78] Schweckendiek W. Two stage closure of cleft palate: Rationale for its use. In: Long-Term Treatment in Cleft Lip Palate with Coordinated Team Approach. Bern: Hans Huber; 1979. p. 254

[79] Schweckendiek W, Doz P. Primary veloplasty: Long-term results without maxillary deformity. A twenty-five year report. The Cleft Palate Journal. 1978;**15**:268-274

[80] Smarius BJ, Breugem CC. Use of early hard palate closure using a vomer flap in cleft lip and palate patients. Journal of Cranio-Maxillo-Facial Surgery. 2016;**44**(8):912-918. DOI: 10.1016/j.jcms.2016.05.011 Epub 2016 May 17

[81] Kehrer B, Universität Bern. Chirurgische Kinderklinik, symposium on late results in the treatment of cleft lip and palate with coordinated team approach. In: Long Term Treatment in Cleft Lip and Palate, with Coordinated Team Approach: Proceedings of the First International Symposium, August 23rd/24th, 1979. Bern: Huber; 1981

[82] Fudalej P, Hortis-Dzierzbicka M, Obloj B, Miller-Drabikowska D, Dudkiewicz Z, Romanowska A. Treatment outcome after one-stage repair in children with complete unilateral cleft lip and palate assessed with the Goslon yardstick. The Cleft Palate-Craniofacial Journal. 2009;**46**(4):374-380. DOI: 10.1597/07-242.1. Epub 2009 Jan 1

[83] Friede H, Lilja J. Dentofacial morphology in adolescent or early adult patients with cleft lip and palate after a treatment regimen that included vomer flap surgery and pushback palatal repair. Scandinavian Journal of Plastic and Reconstructive Surgery and Hand Surgery. 1994;**28**(2):113-121. DOI: 10.3109/02844319409071188

[84] Liao YF, Yang IY, Wang R, Yun C, Huang CS. Two-stage palate repair

with delayed hard palate closure is related to favorable maxillary growth in unilateral cleft lip and palate. Plastic and Reconstructive Surgery. 2010;**125**(5):1503-1510. DOI: 10.1097/PRS.0b013e3181d5132a

[85] Yang IY, Liao YF. The effect of 1-stage versus 2-stage palate repair on facial growth in patients with cleft lip and palate: A review. International Journal of Oral and Maxillofacial Surgery. 2010;**39**(10):945-950. DOI: 10.1016/j.ijom.2010.04.053. Epub 2010 Jul 15

[86] Landheer JA, Breugem CC, van der Molen AB. Fistula incidence and predictors of fistula occurrence after cleft palate repair: Two-stage closure versus one-stage closure. The Cleft Palate-Craniofacial Journal. 2010;**47**:623-630

[87] Willadsen E. Influence of timing of hard palate repair in a two-stage procedure on early speech development in Danish children with cleft palate. The Cleft Palate-Craniofacial Journal. 2012;**49**(5):574-595. DOI: 10.1597/09-120. Epub 2011 Feb 10

[88] Hopper RA, Tse R, Smartt J, Swanson J, Kinter S. Cleft palate repair and velopharyngeal dysfunction. Plastic and Reconstructive Surgery. 2014;**133**(6):852e-864e. DOI: 10.1097/PRS.0000000000000184

[89] Lehner B, Wiltfang J, Strobel-Schwarthoff K, Benz M, Hirschfelder U, Neukam FW. Influence of early hard palate closure in unilateral and bilateral cleft lip and palate on maxillary transverse growth during the first four years of age. The Cleft Palate-Craniofacial Journal. 2003;**40**(2):126-130. DOI: 10.1597/1545-1569_2003_040_0126_ioehpc_2.0.co_2

[90] Randall P, LaRossa DD, Fakhraee SM, Cohen MA. Cleft palate closure at 3 to 7 months of age: A preliminary report. Plastic and Reconstructive Surgery. 1983;**71**(5):624-628. DOI: 10.1097/00006534-198305000-00007

[91] Naidu P, Yao CA, Chong DK, Magee WP 3rd. Cleft palate repair: A history of techniques and variations. Plastic and Reconstructive Surgery. Global Open. 2022;**10**(3):e4019. DOI: 10.1097/GOX.0000000000004019

[92] Bishara SE, Enemark H, Tharp RF. Cephalometric comparisons of the results of the Wardill-Kilner and Von Langenbeck palatoplasties. The Cleft Palate Journal. 1976;**13**:319-329

[93] Sato FRL, da Silva ML, RWF M. Evaluation of two palatoplasty techniques in patients with cleft palate. Otorhinolaryngology-Head and Neck Surgery [Internet]. 2016;**1**(4):1. Available from: https://www.oatext.com/Evaluation-of-two-palatoplasty-techniques-in-patients-with-cleft-palate.php

[94] Bishara SE, Tharp RM. Effects of Von Langenbeck palatoplasty on facial growth. The Angle Orthodontist. 1977;**47**(1):34-41. DOI: 10.1043/0003-3219 (1977)047<0034:EOVLPO>2.0.CO;2

[95] Farzaneh F, Lindman R, Becker M, Hansen K, Svensson H. von Langenbeck procedures at 8 months or Wardill at 18 months for primary repair of cleft palate in adult Swedish patients with unilateral complete cleft lip and palate: A study of facial growth. Scandinavian Journal of Plastic and Reconstructive Surgery and Hand Surgery. 2008;**42**(2):67-76. DOI: 10.1080/02844310701850512

[96] Farzaneh F, Lindman R, Becker M, Hansen K, Svensson H. von Langenbeck procedures at 14 months or Wardill at 18 months for primary repair of cleft palate

in adult Swedish patients with bilateral complete cleft lip and palate: A study of facial growth. Scandinavian Journal of Plastic and Reconstructive Surgery and Hand Surgery. 2009;**43**(4):214-224. DOI: 10.1080/02844310903040789

[97] Semb G. A study of facial growth in patients with unilateral cleft lip and palate treated by the Oslo CLP team. The Cleft Palate-Craniofacial Journal. 1991;**28**(1):1-21; discussion 46-8. DOI: 10.1597/1545-1569_1991_028_0001_asofgi_2.3.co_2

[98] Agrawal K. Cleft palate repair and variations. Indian Journal of Plastic Surgery. 2009;**42**(Suppl.):S102-S109. DOI: 10.4103/0970-0358.57197

[99] van Aalst JA, Kolappa KK, Sadove M. MOC-PSSM CME article: Nonsyndromic cleft palate. Plastic and Reconstructive Surgery. 2008;**121**(Suppl. 1):1-14. DOI: 10.1097/01.prs.0000294706.05898.f3

[100] Furlow LT Jr. Cleft palate repair by double opposing Z-plasty. Plastic and Reconstructive Surgery. 1986;**78**(6):724-738. DOI: 10.1097/00006534-198678060-00002

[101] Braithwaite F, Maurice DG. The importance of the levator palati muscle in cleft palate closure. British Journal of Plastic Surgery. 1968;**21**(1):60-62. DOI: 10.1016/s0007-1226(68)80087-6

[102] Kim YH, Ryu JY, Lee JS, Yang JD, Chung HY, Cho BC, et al. Effect of conservative levator veli palatini dissection on palatoplasty: A retrospective cohort study. Journal of Cranio-Maxillo-Facial Surgery. 2022;**50**(9):699-704. DOI: 10.1016/j.jcms.2022.09.002

[103] Sommerlad BC. Surgery of the cleft palate: Repair using the operating microscope with radical muscle retropositioning–the GostA approach. B-ENT. 2006;**2**(Suppl. 4):32-34

[104] Short Notes in Plastic Surgery. The surgical treatment of cleft palate [Internet]. 2015. Available from: https://shortnotesinplasticsurgery.wordpress.com/2015/07/20/54-the-surgical-treatment-of-cleft-palate/used [Accessed: May 6, 2025]

[105] McGuire E. Cleft lip and palates and breastfeeding. Breastfeeding Review. 2017;**25**(1):17-23

[106] Lehman JA Jr, Douglas BK, Ho WC, Husami TW. One-stage closure of the entire primary palate. Plastic and Reconstructive Surgery. 1990;**86**(4):675-681. DOI: 10.1097/00006534-199010000-00010

[107] Puente Espel J, Hohman MH, Winters R. Cleft palate repair. In: StatPearls [Internet]. Treasure Island (FL): StatPearls Publishing; 2025 [Accessed: July 4, 2023]

[108] Timbang MR, Gharb BB, Rampazzo A, Papay F, Zins J, Doumit G. A systematic review comparing Furlow double-opposing Z-plasty and straight-line intravelar veloplasty methods of cleft palate repair. Plastic and Reconstructive Surgery. 2014;**134**(5):1014-1022. DOI: 10.1097/PRS.0000000000000637

[109] Perry JL, Kuehn DP. Anatomy and physiology of the velopharynx. In: Losee JE, Kirschner RE, editors. Comprehensive Cleft Care. 2nd ed. Boca Raton (FL): CRC Press; 2015. pp. 475-492

[110] Kummer AW. Disorders of resonance and airflow secondary to cleft palate and/or velopharyngeal dysfunction. Seminars in Speech and Language. 2011;**32**(2):141-149. DOI: 10.1055/s-0031-1277716. Epub 2011 Sep 26

[111] Sell D, Mildinhall S, Albery L, Wills AK, Sandy JR, Ness AR. The cleft

care UK study. Part 4: Perceptual speech outcomes. Orthodontics & Craniofacial Research. 2015;**18**(Suppl. 2):36-46. DOI: 10.1111/ocr.12112

[112] Golding-Kushner KJ, Argamaso RV, Cotton RT, et al. Standardization for the reporting of nasopharyngoscopy and multiview videofluoroscopy: A report from an international working group. The Cleft Palate Journal. 1990;**27**:337-347; discussion 347-348

[113] Kummer AW. Speech evaluation for patients with cleft palate. Clinics in Plastic Surgery. 2014;**41**(2):241-251. DOI: 10.1016/j.cps.2013.12.004

[114] Ysunza A, Pamplona M, Femat T, Mayer I, García-Velasco M. Videonasopharyngoscopy as an instrument for visual biofeedback during speech in cleft palate patients. International Journal of Pediatric Otorhinolaryngology. 1997;**41**(3):291-298. DOI: 10.1016/s0165-5876(97)00096-7

[115] Pigott RW, Bensen JF, White FD. Nasendoscopy in the diagnosis of velopharyngeal incompetence. Plastic and Reconstructive Surgery. 1969;**43**(2):141-147. DOI:10.1097/00006534-196902000-00005

[116] Woo AS. Velopharyngeal dysfunction. Seminars in Plastic Surgery. 2012;**26**(4):170-177. DOI: 10.1055/s-0033-1333882

[117] Smetona JT, Naran S, Ford M, Losee JE. What's new in cleft palate and velopharyngeal dysfunction management: An update. Plastic and Reconstructive Surgery. 2024;**154**(2):378e-390e. DOI: 10.1097/PRS.0000000000011312. Epub 2024 Jul 22

[118] Perry JL, Sutton BP, Kuehn DP, Gamage JK. Using MRI for assessing velopharyngeal structures and function. The Cleft Palate-Craniofacial Journal. 2014;**51**(4):476-485. DOI: 10.1597/12-083. Epub 2013 Apr 8. Erratum in: Cleft Palate Craniofac J. 2015 May;52(3):382. DOI: 10.1597/1545-1569-52.3.382

[119] Perry JL, Kollara L, Kuehn DP, Sutton BP, Fang X. Examining age, sex, and race characteristics of velopharyngeal structures in 4- to 9-year old children using magnetic resonance imaging. The Cleft Palate-Craniofacial Journal. 2018;**55**(1):21-34. DOI: 10.1177/1055665617718549. Epub 2017 Dec 14

[120] Perry JL, Williams JL, Snodgrass TD, Sitzman TJ. VPI management in SATB2 syndrome: Use of MRI to evaluate anatomy and physiology in non-cleft VPI. The Cleft Palate-Craniofacial Journal. 2023;**60**(11):1499-1504. DOI: 10.1177/10556656221106888. Epub 2022 Jun 12

[121] Arendt CT, Eichler K, Mack MG, Leithner D, Zhang S, Block KT, et al. Comparison of contrast-enhanced videofluoroscopy to unenhanced dynamic MRI in minor patients following surgical correction of velopharyngeal dysfunction. European Radiology. 2021;**31**(1):76-84. DOI: 10.1007/s00330-020-07098-9. Epub 2020 Aug 1

[122] Marsh JL. Management of velopharyngeal dysfunction: Differential diagnosis for differential management. The Journal of Craniofacial Surgery. 2003;**14**(5):621-628; discussion 629. DOI: 10.1097/00001665-200309000-00004. Erratum in: J Craniofac Surg. 2003 Nov;14(6):936

[123] Shprintzen RJ, Marrinan E. Velopharyngeal insufficiency: Diagnosis and management. Current Opinion in Otolaryngology & Head and Neck Surgery. 2009;**17**(4):302-307. DOI: 10.1097/MOO.0b013e32832cbd6b

[124] Cleft Care Ireland. Secondary Surgery [Internet]. Dublin: Cleft Care Ireland. Available from: https://cleftcareireland.ie/treatment/secondary-surgery; [Accessed: June 29, 2025]

[125] Chauhan JS, Sharma S, Jain D, Junval J. Palatal lengthening by double opposing buccal flaps for surgical correction of velopharyngeal insufficiency in cleft patients. Journal of Cranio-Maxillo-Facial Surgery. 2020;**48**(10):977-984. DOI: 10.1016/j.jcms.2020.08.006. Epub 2020 Sep 3

[126] Haenssler AE, Perry JL, Mann SA, Mann RJ. An MRI case study: The anatomic cleft restoration concept utilizing buccal flaps in a primary palatoplasty [Internet]. FACE. 2021;**2**(2):27325016211006850. DOI: 10.1177/27325016211006850 [Accessed: May 2, 2025]

[127] Mann RJ, Neaman KC, Armstrong SD, Ebner B, Bajnrauh R, Naum S. The double-opposing buccal flap procedure for palatal lengthening. Plastic and Reconstructive Surgery. 2011;**127**(6):2413-2418. DOI: 10.1097/PRS.0b013e3182131d3e

[128] Chiang SN, Fotouhi AR, Grames LM, Skolnick GB, Snyder-Warwick AK, Patel KB. Buccal myomucosal flap repair for velopharyngeal dysfunction. Plastic and Reconstructive Surgery. 2023;**152**(4):842-850. DOI: 10.1097/PRS.0000000000010443. Epub 2023 Mar 21

[129] Whitaker LA, Randall P, Graham WP 3rd, Hamilton RW, Winchester R. A prospective and randomized series comparing superiorly and inferiorly based posterior pharyngeal flaps. The Cleft Palate Journal. 1972;**9**:304-311

[130] Hamlen M. Speech changes after pharyngeal flap surgery. Plastic and Reconstructive Surgery. 1970;**46**(5):437-444. DOI: 10.1097/00006534-197011000-00004

[131] Meek MF, Coert JH, Hofer SO, Goorhuis-Brouwer SM, Nicolai JP. Short-term and long-term results of speech improvement after surgery for velopharyngeal insufficiency with pharyngeal flaps in patients younger and older than 6 years old: 10-year experience. Annals of Plastic Surgery. 2003;**50**(1):13-17. DOI: 10.1097/00000637-200301000-00003

[132] Hogan VM. A clarification of the surgical goals in cleft palate speech and the introduction of the lateral port control (l.p.c.) pharyngeal flap. The Cleft Palate Journal. 1973;**10**:331-345

[133] Arneja JS, Hettinger P, Gosain AK. Through-and-through dissection of the soft palate for high pharyngeal flap inset: A new technique for the treatment of velopharyngeal incompetence in velocardiofacial syndrome. Plastic and Reconstructive Surgery. 2008;**122**(3):845-852. DOI: 10.1097/PRS.0b013e3181811a83

[134] Abdel-Aziz M. Palatopharyngeal sling: A new technique in treatment of velopharyngeal insufficiency. International Journal of Pediatric Otorhinolaryngology. 2008;**72**(2):173-177. DOI: 10.1016/j.ijporl.2007.10.004. Epub 2007 Nov 26

[135] Cheng N, Zhao M, Qi K, Deng H, Fang Z, Song R. A modified procedure for velopharyngeal sphincteroplasty in primary cleft palate repair and secondary velopharyngeal incompetence treatment and its preliminary results. Journal of Plastic, Reconstructive & Aesthetic Surgery. 2006;**59**(8):817-825. DOI: 10.1016/j.bjps.2005.11.006. Epub 2006 Feb 2

[136] Sader R, Zeilhofer HF, Putz R, Horch HH. Levatorplasty, a new technique to treat hypernasality: Anatomical investigations and preliminary clinical results. Journal of Cranio-Maxillo-Facial Surgery. 2001;**29**(3):143-149

[137] Ragab A. Cerclage sphincter pharyngoplasty: A new technique for velopharyngeal insufficiency. International Journal of Pediatric Otorhinolaryngology. 2007;**71**(5):793-800. DOI: 10.1016/j.ijporl.2007.01.020. Epub 2007 Mar 6

[138] Lypka M, Bidros R, Rizvi M, Gaon M, Rubenstein A, Fox D, et al. Posterior pharyngeal augmentation in the treatment of velopharyngeal insufficiency: A 40-year experience. Annals of Plastic Surgery. 2010;**65**(1):48-51. DOI: 10.1097/SAP.0b013e3181c1fec6

[139] Abdali H, Yaribakht M. Assessment of outcomes and complications of posterior pharyngeal wall augmentation with dermal fat graft in patients with velopharyngeal insufficiency (VPI) after primary cleft palate repair: A pilot study. JPRAS Open. 2019;**19**:6-18

[140] Kobayashi S, Mizuno Y, Suzuki M, Yasumura K, Hirakawa T, Fukawa T, et al. Posterior pharyngeal wall augmentation using autologous tiered costal cartilage for velopharyngeal insufficiency. Journal of Plastic, Reconstructive & Aesthetic Surgery. 2022;**75**(6):e1-e6. DOI: 10.1016/j.bjps.2022.01.008. Epub 2022 Jan 20

[141] Bishop A, Hong P, Bezuhly M. Autologous fat grafting for the treatment of velopharyngeal insufficiency: State of the art. Journal of Plastic, Reconstructive & Aesthetic Surgery. 2014;**67**(1):1-8. DOI: 10.1016/j.bjps.2013.09.021. Epub 2013 Sep 20

Section 3

Pediatric Urology

Chapter 5

Disorders of Sex Development and Androgen Insensitivity Syndrome

Ilhama Jafarli

Abstract

When gonadal, anatomical, or chromosomal sex development deviates from typical patterns, resulting in discordance between phenotypic presentations of sex traits and chromosomal sex, a complex range of illnesses known as Disorders of Sex Development (DSDs) may occur. Depending on the severity, it could appear at birth, during puberty, or sometimes go undiagnosed until later in life. Since DSDs defy binary concepts of male and female biological traits, a deep understanding of scientific fields and societal settings is required. DSDs have a variety of biological causes, including the developmental abnormalities, hormone imbalances, and genetic mutations. Atypical numbers of sex chromosomes cause chromosomal abnormalities, including Turner syndrome (45,X) and Klinefelter syndrome (47,XXY). A sex development pathway may also be impacted by gonadal dysgenesis, a disorder in which the gonads do not develop normally. Hormonal factors are important; for instance, those with XY chromosomes who are resistant to male hormones develop Androgen Insensitivity Syndrome (AIS), which results in external traits that are traditionally associated with women. People with a 46, XY karyotype who have Androgen Insensitivity Syndrome (AIS), a disease of sex development (DSD), have varying degrees of androgen resistance due to mutations in the androgen receptor gene. Complete AIS (CAIS) is characterized by the presence of female external genitalia and undescended testes; however, in Partial (PAIS) and Mild (MAIS) forms, masculinization is partially preserved. This condition is a true example of the complex interaction between genetic, hormonal, and anatomical sex development. Diagnosis consists of chromosomal analysis, hormone profiling, imaging, and molecular testing for AR gene mutations.

Keywords: androgen receptors, androgen insensitivity syndrome, disorders of sex development, sex ambiguity, androgens

1. Introduction

A series of illnesses known as disorders of sex development (DSDs) occur when gonadal, anatomical, or chromosomal sex development is abnormal, resulting in a divergence between phenotypic and chromosomal sex traits. These diseases can range from minor to severe and may show up at birth or during puberty. Traditional conceptions of male and female biological characteristics may be challenged by the ways that DSDs impact sexual development. They frequently dictate complicated relationships between environmental, hormonal, and genetic variables.

People with XX chromosomes typically have female reproductive organs and genitalia, whereas people with XY chromosomes develop male reproductive organs. However, this process is interrupted at some stage of development in people with DSDs, resulting in differences in sexual characteristics. These differences can be recognised later in life, during puberty, or at birth.

Essential Features of DSD:

- Chromosomal variations: Conditions like Turner syndrome (45,X) or Klinefelter syndrome (47,XXY) are examples of deviations from the normal XX (female) or XY (male) chromosomal patterns.

- Gonadal variations: It is possible that the gonads—the ovaries or testes—will not develop normally in either the male or female forms. People may, for example, have gonads that are not differentiated or a combination of ovarian and testicular tissue.

- Phenotypic variations: Chromosomal or gonadal sex may not correspond with their outward sexual traits, such as their genitalia.

1.1 Chromosomal sex determination (XX vs. XY)

Sex determination starts with chromosomes. Females normally have XX chromosomes, while males have XY chromosomes. The presence of the Y chromosome triggers male differentiation through the *SRY* gene, which activates the development of testes. In the absence of the SRY gene, gonads grow into ovaries, regardless of the presence of the Y chromosome, as seen in conditions like *Swyer syndrome*.

1.2 Gonadal differentiation (ovaries vs. testes)

Once chromosomal sex is confirmed, gonads develop into either testes or ovaries. In XY individuals, the SRY gene leads the formation of testes, which produce testosterone and *anti-Müllerian hormone (AMH)*. Testosterone stimulates male internal structures (e.g., vas deferens), and AMH prevents the formation of female organs. In XX individuals, the absence of SRY directs to ovarian development, with oestrogen driving the formation of female reproductive organs (e.g., uterus, fallopian tubes).

1.3 Hormonal influences (androgens and oestrogens)

Testosterone and masculinization: Testosterone is important for the development of male internal structures. It stimulates the development of the Wolffian ducts into male structures such as the epididymis, vas deferens, and seminal vesicles. In the presence of dihydrotestosterone (DHT), a more potent form of testosterone, the external genitalia differentiate into male characteristics, including the penis and scrotum.

Absence of testosterone and feminization: In the absence of testosterone (as seen in females or in conditions where there is androgen insensitivity), the Wolffian ducts regress, and the Müllerian ducts differentiate into female structures like the uterus, fallopian tubes, and upper two thirds of the vagina. Oestrogen produced by the ovaries plays a role in the development of female external genitalia, such as the clitoris, labia, and vaginal opening.

2. Embryological development of sexual characteristics

The embryological development of sexual characteristics is a highly regulated process involving complex exchanges between chromosomes, genes, and hormones. The interplay of these factors determines whether an individual will develop male or female characteristics, both internally and externally.

However, when this process is interrupted, it can result in Disorders of Sex Development (DSDs), which highlight the variability and complexity of human sexual development. Understanding the underlying mechanisms of sexual differentiation and the factors that contribute to DSDs is vital not only for medical diagnosis and management but also for fostering greater acceptance of the natural diversity in human biology.

This begins with the sex chromosomes and is influenced by the *SRY* gene, which is key for male differentiation, and other genes like *SOX9* for testes development. In females, the absence of SRY allows ovarian differentiation through the *WNT4* gene.

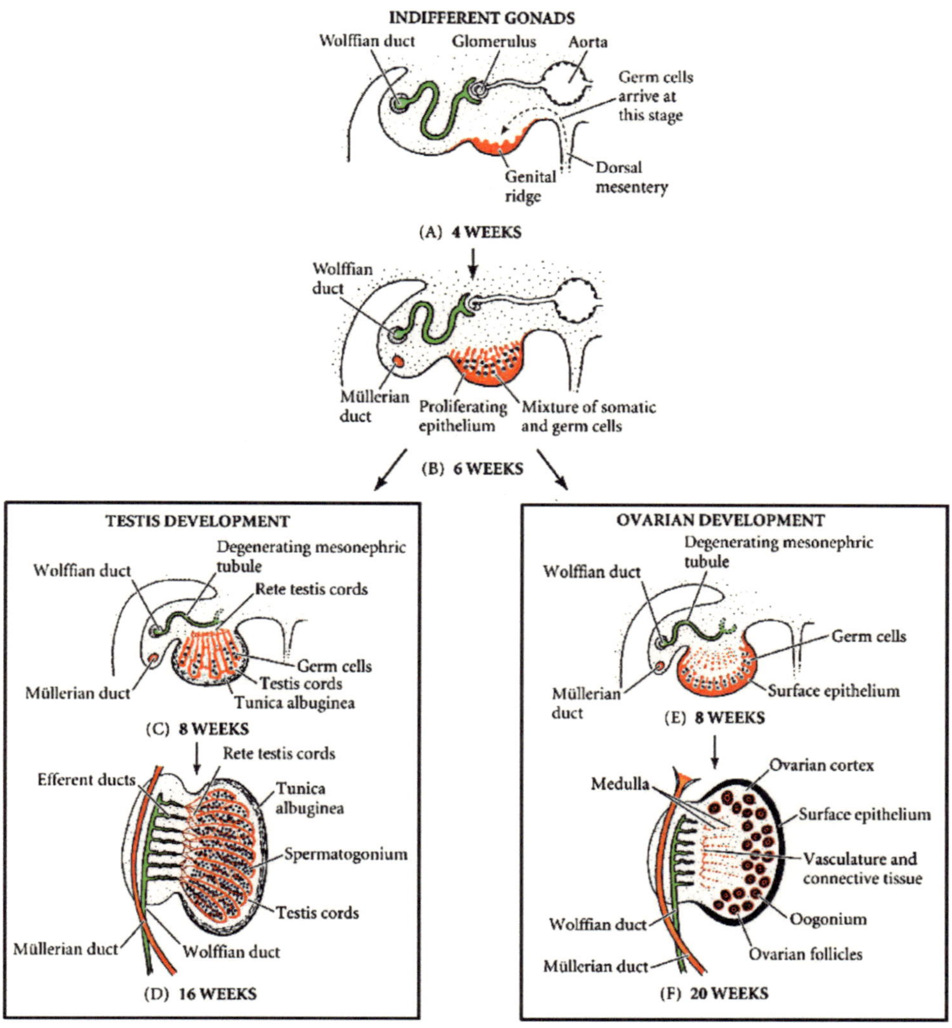

Figure 1.
Embryonic development of gonads: testes and ovaries. Adapted from work by Gilbert Scott F., licenced under CC BY 3.0, via Wikimedia Commons.

Hormones like testosterone and oestrogen drive the formation of internal and external genitalia, leading to sex development.

As a result, the external sex features do not match what the sex chromosomes would normally suggest. Some neonates show clear differences right away, while others only appeal during puberty or later. Because DSDs can be mild, moderate, or severe, they often complicate familiar ideas about what it means to be biologically male or female. Most experts agree that gene activity, hormone levels, and even some outside factors work together to produce these variations.

Under normal circumstances, people with two X chromosomes form female genitalia and reproductive organs, whereas those with one X and one Y chromosome develop male structures. When the sequence runs into trouble, however, the resulting anatomy can fall anywhere along the range between the two extremes. Because of this, an anomaly might be noticeable at birth, become evident during the anticipated changes of puberty, or surface later when reproduction plans arise (**Figure 1**).

3. DSD's key aspects

1. *Medical implications*: The presence of a DSD can present complex disorders, requiring specialised diagnostic approaches, treatment plans, and long-term management. This often involves endocrinologists, genetic counsellors, surgeons, urologists and psychologists to address the physical, hormonal, and psychological aspects of the condition.

2. *Genetic insights*: Studying DSDs has provided valuable insights into the genetic, hormonal, and developmental pathways that control sexual differentiation. Understanding the mutations and regulatory mechanisms that lead to DSDs requires refined knowledge in genetics, endocrinology, and developmental biology.

3. *Psychosocial considerations*: DSDs can have significant psychological and social impact on affected individuals, especially in terms of gender identity and the societal expectations associated with male and female roles. Early intervention and comprehensive care are crucial to address not just the physical aspects, but also the emotional and social well-being of individuals with DSDs.

4. *Ethical and societal issues*: DSDs raise important ethical questions, particularly regarding early medical or surgical interventions to assign gender at birth. There is growing recognition of the importance of informed consent and allowing individuals to have agency over choices about their bodies and gender identity, especially as they reach adulthood.

5. *Reproductive health*: DSDs can affect fertility, causing reproductive health problems that need to be addressed as part of a comprehensive care plan. Some individuals with DSDs would require assisted reproductive services if they wish to have biological children.

6. *Human diversity*: DSDs challenge the binary concepts of male and female, highlighting the natural variability in human biology and supporting a broad understanding of gender. This view can help reduce stigma and increase acceptance of individuals with variations in sexual development (**Table 1**).

Category	Anomalies in sex determination (chromosomes and gonads)	Anomalies in sex differentiation (hormones and enzymes)
A. Without sex ambiguity (usually)	1. Gonadal Dysgenesis (a) Ovarian Agenesis (b) Gonadal Dysgenesis with Chromosomal and/or Phenotypic Alteration (Turner Syndrome) (c) Ovarian Dysgenesis or Hypoplasia	1. Testicular Dysgenesis (XY) (a) Dysgenetic Male Ps or Partial Gonadal Dysgenesis (b) Mixed Gonadal Dysgenesis
	2. Variants of Gonadal Dysgenesis (a) Mosaic Variants (b) Structural Abnormalities of the Second Sex Chromosome (c) Pure Gonadal Dysgenesis (Swyer Syndrome)	2. Deficiencies in the Testicle Itself or its Secretions (1) Embryonic Testicular Regression (Anorchia) (2) Disorders of Androgen Production (MAD due to enzyme deficiencies)
	3. Triple X Constitution and Other Polysomies	3. Mutations in the NR5A1 Gene/SF-1
	4. Sex Reversal (Males XX)	4. Defects in Androgenic Action or Androgen Insensitivity Syndrome (AIS) - 5α-reductase deficiency or androgen receptor function disorders
	5. Klinefelter Syndrome (Males)	5. Hormone Therapy, Iatrogenic
	6. Dysgenetic Infertility	6. Aromatase Deficiency (P450arom)
B. With sex ambiguity (usually)		1. Congenital Adrenal Hyperplasia in Female/ Adrenogenital Syndrome (1) 17-α-Hydroxylase Deficiency (CYP17A1) (2) Cytochrome P450-Oxidoreductase Deficiency (PORD) (3) 21-Hydroxylase Deficiency (P450c21) (4) 11-β-Hydroxylase Deficiency (P450c11)
		2. True Hermaphroditism or Ovotesticular Disorders (OT-DSD)
		3. Maternal Virilizing Tumour
C. Without Ps		1. Congenital Hypogonadotropic Hypogonadism (CHH) - (Kallmann Syndrome, Males and Females)

PS: pseudohermaphroditism; MAD: male with androgen deficiency; FAE: female with androgen excess; DSDs: disorders of sex development; OT: ovotesticular; AIS: androgen insensitivity syndromes; CYP: Cytochrome P450.

Table 1.
The new nomenclature for the classification of disorders of sex development proposed by Pedro Acien and Maribel Acien [1].

4. Androgen insensitivity syndrome (AIS) and sexual differentiation

One of the key examples of a DSD is *Androgen Insensitivity Syndrome (AIS)*, a condition in which an individual who is genetically male (with XY chromosomes) has a partial or complete inability to respond to male sex hormones, known as androgens. This results in the formation of predominantly female physical characteristics, despite the presence of male chromosomes. AIS can be classified into three main types: complete androgen insensitivity syndrome (CAIS), partial androgen insensitivity syndrome (PAIS) and mild androgen insensitivity syndrome (MAIS), depending on the degree of insensitivity to androgens.

AIS represents a clear illustration of how genetic and hormonal factors interact in the process of sexual differentiation. Understanding AIS, its causes, and its consequences is crucial for proper diagnosis, management, and support for individuals affected by this disorder. This summary analyses the biological mechanisms behind AIS, its clinical presentation, diagnostic approaches, the social and psychological impact on individuals with DSDs like AIS.

5. Understanding androgen insensitivity syndrome (AIS)

Androgen Insensitivity Syndrome (AIS) is a rare X-linked genetic disorder characterised by the impaired ability of people with a 46, XY karyotype to respond to androgens, the male sex hormones. This condition is a result of mutations in the androgen receptor (AR) gene located at Xq12, which is responsible for the normal development of male sexual features. These mutations prevent the androgen receptors from functioning properly, thus impairing virilization and triggering the development of a predominantly female phenotype despite the presence of male chromosomes. The condition's clinical presentation varies greatly based on the type and severity of the androgen receptor dysfunction.

6. Genetics and pathophysiology of AIS

AIS is mainly caused by mutations in the *AR gene* (androgen receptor gene), located on the X chromosome. The AR gene encodes the androgen receptor (AR), a protein that is responsible for binding androgens (such as testosterone and dihydrotestosterone). When the AR gene is mutated, the androgen receptor becomes defective or absent, blocking the proper binding and action of androgens. This results in a lack of androgen sensitivity, which affects the development of male sexual characteristics during intrauterine life and postnatal development.

Approximately 70% of AIS mutations are maternally inherited, while the remaining 30% arise de novo. The AR gene mutations may happen in different regions, including the *N-terminal domain (NTD)* and the *ligand-binding domain (LBD)*. Mutations in the NTD are more likely to result in *Complete Androgen Insensitivity Syndrome (CAIS)*, while mutations in the LBD can lead to either *CAIS* or *Partial Androgen Insensitivity Syndrome (PAIS)*, proportional to the severity of receptor dysfunction [2].

The *AR gene* plays an important role in male sexual differentiation by enabling the body to respond to androgens. Mutations in the AR gene give rise to varying degrees of androgen insensitivity. The mutations can be either complete or partial, depending on the degree to which the receptor is non functional or defective. The AR gene mutations could cause either a reduced number of functional receptors or a complete absence of functional receptors on target tissues, especially those involved in sexual differentiation, such as the genitalia and reproductive organs.

In patients with AIS, these mutations inhibit the androgen receptors from binding testosterone and other androgens, causing the failure of masculinization of the external genitalia and other male sexual characteristics. The effect of these mutations can fluctuate, leading to different clinical presentations based on the severity of receptor dysfunction. Mutations in the AR gene are typically inherited in an X-linked recessive manner, which means the condition is more common in males, but females can also be carriers and show mild forms of the condition in rare cases.

Mutations in the AR gene impair the ability of androgen receptors to interact with androgens. Normally, when testosterone or its more potent form, dihydrotestosterone (DHT), binds to the androgen receptor, it activates a cascade of intracellular signalling that leads to the development of male secondary sexual characteristics. This process involves the formation of male external genitalia (such as the penis and scrotum) and the internal reproductive organs (such as the prostate and seminal vesicles).

In AIS, the defective or absent androgen receptor means that testosterone cannot utilise its effects on the developing tissues. In *Complete Androgen Insensitivity Syndrome (CAIS)*, the androgen receptor is non functional, and in *Partial and Mild Androgen Insensitivity Syndrome (PAIS and MAIS)*, the receptor may still have some ability to bind androgens, but it is not fully functional. This difference in receptor functionality describes the variation in the phenotype of individuals with AIS.

The lack of androgen sensitivity in AIS is an immediate consequence of mutations that prevent androgen receptors from responding to testosterone and other androgens. Normally, testosterone produced by the testes during foetal development plays a crucial role in the masculinization of the internal and external genitalia. However, in AIS, due to the defective androgen receptors, these hormonal signals are not predictable or acted upon by the target tissues.

This failure in androgen receptor signalling leads to the development of external genitalia that appears female, despite the presence of XY chromosomes. For example, people with CAIS will often have a typical female external appearance (vagina, clitoris, labia), even though their internal gonads are testes. However, because the internal testes do not respond to the hormones, the Müllerian ducts (which normally develop into female internal genitalia such as the uterus and fallopian tubes) regress, blocking the formation of female reproductive organs.

Furthermore, the absence of androgen signalling during puberty results in the failure to develop male secondary sexual characteristics such as facial hair, deepening of the voice, and increased muscle mass, while female secondary sexual characteristics like breast development may still occur. This discrepancy between chromosomal sex (XY) and phenotypic sex (female) is a hallmark feature of AIS.

7. Types of AIS

AIS is classified into three main types based on the degree of androgen insensitivity:

Complete Androgen Insensitivity Syndrome (CAIS) is the most severe form of AIS, where the androgen receptor is totally non functional. As a result, individuals with CAIS do not respond to androgens at all. These people typically develop normal female external genitalia, including a clitoris, labia, and a shallow vaginal opening. They also have testes that remain undescended (not in the scrotum) due to the lack of androgen signalling. While individuals with CAIS have XY chromosomes and internal testes, they do not develop male genitalia, and their sexual characteristics are exclusively female.

CAIS is often diagnosed during adolescence or early adulthood when a lack of menstruation or the presence of inguinal (groin) hernias (due to undescended testes) provokes further investigation. Individuals with CAIS typically have a normal female gender identity and are raised as females.

Partial Androgen Insensitivity Syndrome (PAIS) is characterised by a partial inability to respond to androgens. In PAIS, the androgen receptor is partially functional, granting for some androgen action. This means that individuals with PAIS may have ambiguous genitalia that may not clearly look like male or female genitalia, leading to a more complex phenotype. The degree of androgen sensitivity in PAIS can vary, and individuals may present with a range of external genitalia, from mostly male to predominantly female features.

In PAIS, incomplete masculinization of external genitalia is mainly observed, leading to conditions such as hypospadias (a condition where the urethral opening is on the underside of the penis), micropenis, or incomplete scrotal development. Some of them may also experience gynecomastia (breast development) during puberty due to an imbalance between testosterone and oestrogen.

Mild Androgen Insensitivity Syndrome is the mildest form of AIS. This condition have only a slight reduction in androgen sensitivity. They may show mild degrees of masculinization and typically present with male external genitalia, despite some may have slight abnormalities such as mild hypospadias or reduced fertility [3]. This often goes unnoticed until later in life when fertility issues are discovered.

Androgen receptor (AR) expression in the foreskin has been studied to understand its role in hypospadias. Systematic review analysed 8 studies, with conflicting findings: four reported increased AR expression in hypospadias, three found decreased levels, and one showed no difference. AR expression was mostly higher in stromal tissue than in the epithelium [4].

8. Clinical presentation and diagnosis

The clinical presentation of AIS can range from a complete feminization of the external genitalia (as seen in CAIS) to ambiguous or underdeveloped male genitalia (as seen in PAIS). In some cases, the diagnosis is not made until adolescence or adulthood, particularly in cases where CAIS may present with primary amenorrhea or sparse body hair [5]. For MAIS, the condition may only be recognised in adulthood when concerns such as infertility or gynecomastia arise.

The *diagnosis* of AIS often begins with a clinical evaluation, including a thorough physical examination and a review of the medical history. Diagnostic investigations include:

- *Karyotyping*: This confirms the 46, XY chromosomal pattern.
- *DNA sequencing*: This identifies mutations in the AR gene.
- *Hormonal evaluations*: Measuring levels of testosterone and oestrogen can provide insights into the androgen sensitivity and gonadal function.
- *Ultrasonography/MRI scans*: These imaging modalities can be used to identify the presence of undescended testes, a common feature in AIS.

Early diagnosis is vital for the management of AIS, as it allows for appropriate interventions such as gonadectomy (removal of undescended testes), hormone replacement therapy, and psychological support. Genetic counselling is also recommended to help affected individuals and their families understand the genetic basis of the disorder and the implications for future generations.

Whole Exome Sequencing (WES) was used to identify the cause of DSD in a consanguineous family with two 46, XY females exhibiting normal external genitalia. Sanger sequencing validated the candidate variant. Bioinformatics analyses, including molecular dynamics and docking simulations, expected the structural effect of the novel hemizygous p.L763V variant in the AR gene, consistent with X-linked recessive inheritance [6].

Pelvic MRI showed elliptic T1/T2 signal nodules in the bilateral inguinal region, absence of uterus and ovaries, and a short blind-ending vagina. Karyotype analysis revealed 46, XY, supporting a initial diagnosis of CAIS. Laparoscopic bilateral gonadectomy was performed, and histology confirmed dysplastic testicular tissue without malignancy. Sanger sequencing identified a novel hemizygous nonsense mutation, c.927 T > G (p.Tyr309*), in exon 1 of the AR gene [7].

9. Management of AIS

The management of AIS involves a multidisciplinary approach, addressing both the physical and psychological aspects of the disorder. The goal of treatment is to ensure optimal sexual development, fertility options (when possible), and psychological well-being. Management options differ depending on the type of AIS and the severity of symptoms, but common interventions include:

1. *Gonadectomy*:

   As individuals with AIS do not have functional male or female reproductive organs, gonadectomy is usually recommended to prevent the potential risk of gonadal tumours, which may arise from undescended testes. The timing of gonadectomy should be carefully considered, balancing the need for early intervention with the potential psychological impact.

2. *Hormone replacement therapy (HRT):*

   Hormone therapy is an essential component of managing AIS. In CAIS, oestrogen replacement therapy is initiated to promote the development of secondary sexual characteristics such as breast development and the maintenance of bone health. In cases of PAIS or MAIS, testosterone therapy could be administered, although the response can vary depending on the degree of androgen sensitivity.

3. *Creation of a functional vagina*:

   For individuals with CAIS, creating a functional vagina may be necessary, particularly if they desire vaginal intercourse. This can be achieved surgically such as vaginal dilation or construction of a neovagina.

4. *Psychological support and counselling*:

   Diagnosis of AIS can be psychologically distressing, especially for those with gender identity concerns or those dealing with the stigma associated with the condition. A holistic approach that includes psychological counselling is fundamental to support their emotional well-being. The involvement of a multidisciplinary team (MDT) of healthcare providers, including endocrinologists, genetic counsellors, psychologists, urologists and surgeons, is vital for the comprehensive care of individuals with AIS.

5. *Genetic counselling*:

Since AIS is an X-linked condition, genetic counselling is highly recommended for families affected by AIS. This helps families understand the inheritance pattern, the risks of passing the condition on to offspring, and the implications of genetic testing for other family members (**Figure 2**).

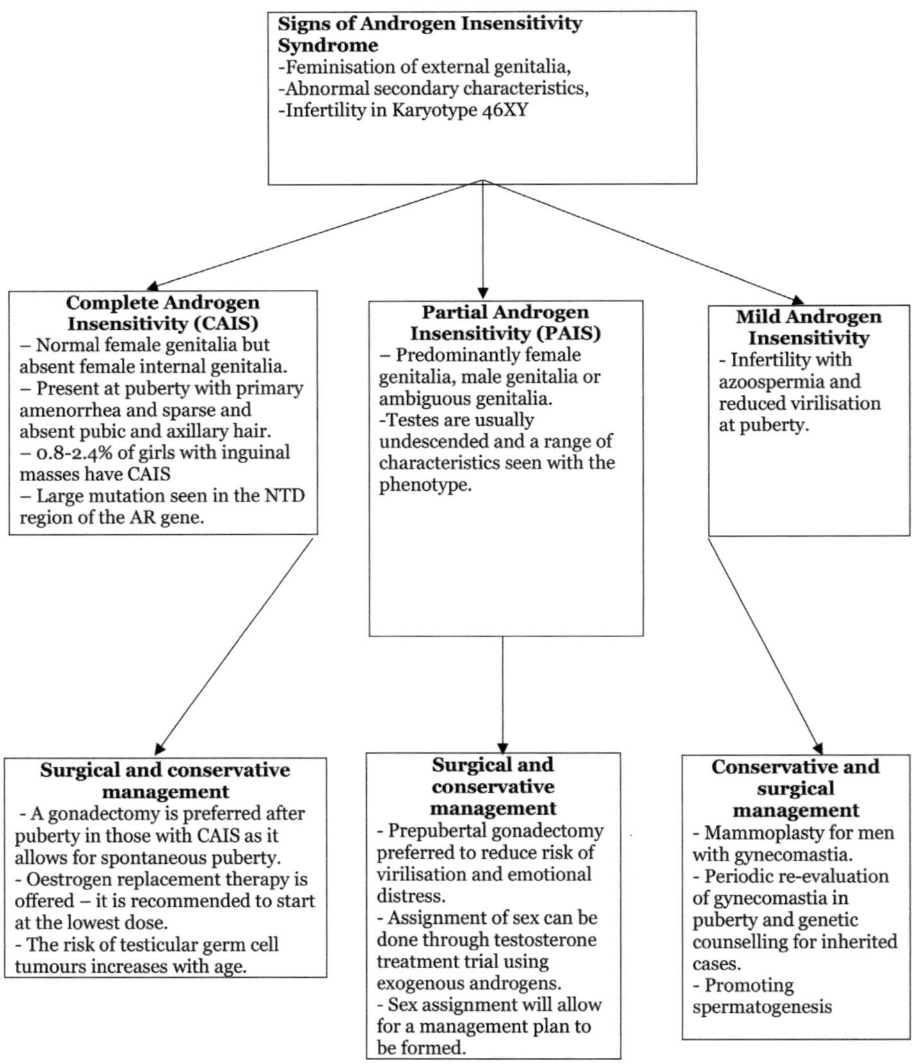

Figure 2.
Diagnosis and management of children with androgen insensitivity syndrome by I Jafarli [8].

One of the common findings in Partial Androgen Insensitivity is the presence of inguinal hernias, as seen in this cohort, where patients presented with inguinal swelling or reducible hernias that prompted further investigation and ultimately led to the diagnosis of Partial Androgen Insensitivity Syndrome (PAIS).

All four patients presented with inguinal hernias, with partially or fully reducible swellings noticed on clinical examination. Cases 1 and 2 presented within the first month of life, an age at which inguinal hernias in phenotypically female or undervirilized infants frequently prompt investigation into disorders of sex development (DSD). Case 3 was noted to have partial scrotal transposition, a form of atypical genital development where the scrotal folds are asymmetrically positioned. Case 4 had an intraoperative discovery of persistent Müllerian structures (uterus and fallopian tubes), raising suspicion for Persistent Müllerian Duct Syndrome (PMDS). However, follow-up testing (AMH and AMH receptor gene analysis) excluded PMDS as the primary diagnosis.

All patients had a 46,XY karyotype, confirming a male chromosomal pattern despite undervirilization.

Hormonal profile demonstrated age-appropriate testosterone and dihydrotestosterone (DHT) levels, indicating intact androgen biosynthesis. Luteinizing Hormone (LH) and Follicle Stimulating Hormone (FSH) were elevated in all cases, suggestive of androgen resistance due to impaired negative feedback on the hypothalamic-pituitary-gonadal axis. Anti-Müllerian Hormone (AMH) was present in all cases, including Case 4; however, Case 4 had retained Müllerian structures, leading to further evaluation.

Ultrasound and laparoscopy confirmed absence or intra-abdominal location of testes, with no Müllerian structures except in Case 4. Case 4 underwent AMH receptor gene testing (AMHR2), which was negative, ruling out PMDS as a standalone diagnosis. The presence of Müllerian remnants was attributed to a variant presentation of PAIS, likely due to AR mutation-related partial resistance during critical embryological regression of the Müllerian system.

AR gene sequencing identified pathogenic missense mutations in the ligand-binding domain (LBD) in all four cases. The mutations were predicted to impair androgen-receptor complex activation, which is critical for genital masculinization during embryogenesis. Based on clinical presentation, hormonal profile, imaging, and molecular testing, all four cases were diagnosed with Partial Androgen Insensitivity Syndrome (PAIS).

All patients underwent inguinal hernia repair and bilateral orchidopexy during infancy to prevent complications such as torsion or malignancy, and to facilitate monitoring of gonadal function and malignancy risk. In Case 4, long-term planning included laparoscopic excision of Müllerian remnants due to potential risk of infection, malignancy, or psychosocial implications in later life.

Gonadectomy was deferred until post-pubertal age in accordance with international guidelines, to allow for spontaneous pubertal development, particularly breast development in PAIS, and to preserve endogenous hormone production. Sex assignment decisions were carefully guided by genital phenotype, potential for pubertal development, parental input, and anticipated psychosocial outcomes.

Individualised plans were created for long term care, addressing future needs such as hormone replacement therapy (HRT), fertility counselling, psychological support, and transition to adult services (**Figure 3**).

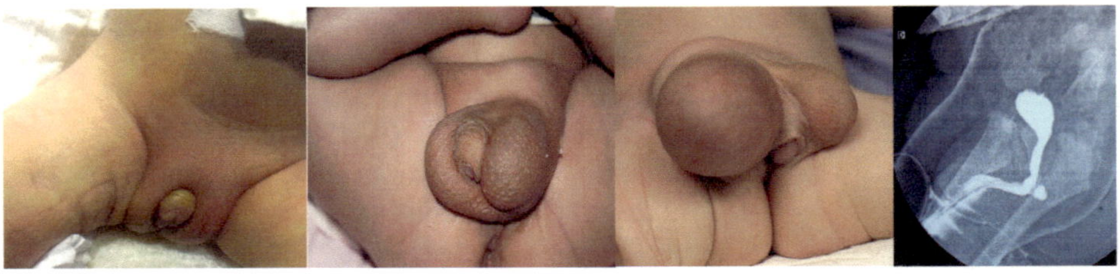

Case 1. Case 2. Case 3. Case 4.

Figure 3.
Clinical spectrum of Androgen Insensitivity Syndrome (AIS)

10. Conclusion

Disorders of Sex Development represent a group of conditions characterised by atypical development of chromosomal, gonadal or anatomical sex, resulting in discrepancies between genetic, gonadal, and phenotypic sex. These conditions are usually evident at birth, during puberty, or later in life, and they range in severity, often challenging traditional understanding of male and female biological traits.

Androgen Insensitivity Syndrome is a complex condition that lies at the intersection of genetics, endocrinology, urology, and human development. It results from mutations in the androgen receptor gene, leading to a partial or complete inability of the body to respond to androgens.

Clinically, AIS manifests across a spectrum, ranging from the typical female external genitalia despite an XY karyotype (Complete AIS), to those with varying degrees of undervirilization (Partial AIS). Diagnosis often occurs during investigations for primary amenorrhea, inguinal hernia in girls, or disorders of sexual development in neonates. A comprehensive understanding of both the biological basis and clinical presentation of AIS is important for accurate diagnosis and effective management. Early diagnosis, coupled with an individualised, multidisciplinary care approach, is vital in supporting both physical health and emotional well-being.

Management strategies must be tailored to each patient's specific needs and involve endocrinologists, geneticists, paediatric surgeons, urologists and mental health professionals. The decision-making process should be guided by clear communication, informed consent, and respect for the patient's autonomy.

Looking ahead, continued research is vital to further unravel the molecular mechanisms behind AIS and to refine diagnostic and treatment protocols. Advancements in genetic testing and hormone therapy hold promise for more accurate and earlier diagnoses. Equally important is the commitment to education-both for healthcare providers and the public-to reduce stigma and promote understanding of disorders of sex development.

Finally, the psychosocial dimensions of AIS must not be disregarded. An empathetic approach that prioritises mental health, body image, gender identity, and peer support is essential. Building a supportive environment where individuals with AIS feel seen, respected, and empowered is just as significant as the clinical care they receive. In embracing a universal model of care, we move toward a future where individuals with AIS can thrive both medically and emotionally.

DOI: http://dx.doi.org/10.5772/intechopen.1013383

Author details

Ilhama Jafarli[1,2]

1 Chelsea and Westminster Hospital, London, United Kingdom

2 Institute of Molecular Biology and Biotechnologies, Baku, Azerbaijan

*Address all correspondence to: ilhama.jafarli@nhs.net

References

[1] Acién P, Acién MI. The history of female genital tract malformation classifications and proposal of an updated system. Human Reproduction Update. 2011;**17**(5):693-705. DOI: 10.1093/humupd/dmr021

[2] Lanciotti L, Cofini M, Leonardi A, Bertozzi M, Penta L, Esposito S. Different clinical presentations and management in complete androgen insensitivity syndrome (CAIS). International Journal of Environmental Research and Public Health. 2019;**16**(7):1268. DOI: 10.3390/ijerph16071268

[3] Bianca S, Cataliotti A, Bartoloni G, Torrente I, Barrano B, Boemi G, et al. Prenatal diagnosis of androgen insensitivity syndrome. Fetal Diagnosis and Therapy. 2009;**26**(3):167-169. DOI: 10.1159/000251712

[4] Oladipo FT, Jafarli I, Huseynova İ, Reynolds HE. Androgen receptor expression in the foreskin of children born with hypospadias: A systematic review. Pediatric Surgery International. 2025;**41**:301. DOI: 10.1007/s00383-025-06205-5

[5] Nezzo M, De Visschere P, T'sjoen G, Weyers S, Villeirs G. Role of imaging in the diagnosis and management of complete androgen insensitivity syndrome in adults. eRadiology. 2013;**2013**:158484. DOI: 10.1155/2013/158484

[6] Aghaei S, Parvizpour S, Farrokhi E, Molavi N, Hoseinzadeh M, Tabatabaiefar MA. Characterization of a novel androgen receptor gene variant identified in an Iranian family with complete androgen insensitivity syndrome (CAIS): A molecular dynamics simulation study. Journal of Biomolecular Structure & Dynamics. 2023;**41**(19):9850-9864. DOI: 10.5582/irdr.2023.01024

[7] Wang K, Wang Q, Chen J, Wang Y, Ma X. Case report: A novel nonsense mutation in the androgen receptor gene causing the complete androgen insensitivity syndrome. Reproductive Sciences. 2022;**29**(9):2659-2663

[8] Jafarli I, John B, Fahmy M, Syed M, Mishra P, Huseynova I. Diagnosis and management of androgen insensitivity syndrome in children. Global Journal of Pediatrics and Neonatal Care. 2023;**4**:000584. DOI: 10.33552/GJPNC.2023.04.000584

Chapter 6

Robotic-Assisted Laparoscopic Pyeloplasty

Jason Yang, Aidan Weitzner and Chad Crigger

Abstract

Strategies and techniques for minimally invasive pyeloplasty in the pediatric population will be reviewed. Included in this will be a thorough assessment and evaluation as well as technical considerations for multiport and emerging single port robotic-assisted surgery. As the robotic platform adopts more widespread usage, the minimal threshold at which a robotic approach may be attempted trends lower, allowing surgeons to use this surgical advantage in the properly selected patient. Challenges with port placement or redo pyeloplasty require careful consideration and will be explored in this most up-to-date chapter synthesizing the existing literature and providing a roadmap for pyeloplasty in the future.

Keywords: pyeloplasty, minimally invasive, robotic, laparoscopic, ureteral reconstruction

1. Introduction

Pyeloplasty is an essential surgical intervention for the treatment of uretero-pelvic junction obstruction (UPJO), a condition in which the normal flow of urine from the kidney to the ureter is impaired. This obstruction can lead to progressive hydronephrosis, recurrent urinary tract infections, pain, and ultimately, deterioration of renal function if left untreated. UPJO is identified as the most prevalent cause of hydronephrosis and affects both children and adults. The diagnosis and evaluation of UPJO have evolved considerably with advancements in imaging techniques, enabling earlier and more accurate detection. Over time, the management of UPJO has shifted from open surgical repair to minimally invasive techniques, including laparoscopic and robotic-assisted pyeloplasty, which offer the benefits of reduced postoperative discomfort, shorter hospital stays, quicker recovery, and favorable cosmetic outcomes. Despite these advancements, patient selection and management of complex cases continue to pose important clinical challenges. This chapter aims to provide a clear, comprehensive overview of pyeloplasty, outlining its indications, diagnostic workup, surgical techniques, evolving innovations, and considerations in special patient populations, to inform both experienced clinicians and readers less familiar.

2. Epidemiology and etiology

UPJO is the most common cause of postnatal hydronephrosis, with an estimated incidence of 1 in 1250 live births and a male predominance of approximately 2.7:1 [1]. UPJO refers to a structural or anatomical narrowing at the junction between the renal pelvis and proximal ureter, impairing the normal outflow of urine from the kidney. This results in increased pressure within the renal collecting system and subsequent hydronephrosis. Urinary stasis can increase the risk of infections and contribute to renal functional decline due to elevated intratubular pressure and parenchymal damage [2, 3]. Although UPJO can be either congenital or acquired (due to instrumentation, nephrolithiasis, or trauma), the majority of cases in the pediatric population are congenital [4, 5].

Etiologically, UPJO is categorized into intrinsic and extrinsic causes (**Figure 1**). Intrinsic UPJO, which accounts for most cases, results from structural or functional abnormalities within the uteropelvic junction itself that impair urine flow [6]. This is typically due to a segment of ureter with defective peristalsis, caused by inadequate development of smooth muscle fibers, focal fibrosis, or aberrant innervation. Intrinsic UPJO is more common in newborns and infants. In contrast, extrinsic UPJO involves external mechanical compression of the ureteropelvic junction by adjacent structures, most commonly by aberrant crossing vessels, such as a lower pole renal artery [7, 8]. Extrinsic obstruction is more frequently diagnosed in childhood and adolescence.

The natural history of UPJO is variable. Some cases resolve spontaneously; two-thirds of cases identified antenatally resolve within the first year [9]. More than half of patients with mild hydronephrosis also achieve spontaneous resolution [10]. However, other cases progress and ultimately require surgical correction. Clinical decision-making is influenced by the severity of hydronephrosis, the presence of symptoms (e.g., pain or recurrent infection), and functional integrity of the affected kidney [11].

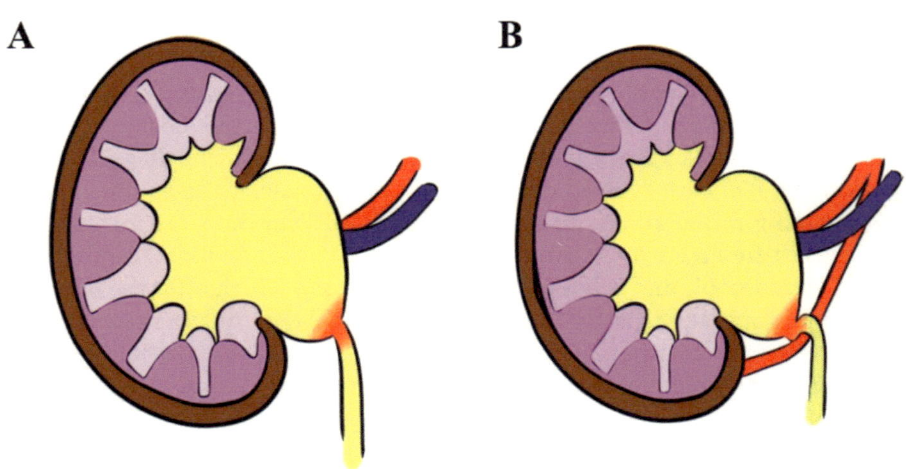

Figure 1.
Etiology of UPJO can be divided into (A) intrinsic causes and (B) extrinsic causes, typically from an aberrant crossing vessel.

3. Patient presentation, diagnosis, and work-up

Historically, intrinsic UPJO in infants often presented with a palpable flank mass on physical examination [12]. However, with the widespread adoption of routine prenatal ultrasonography, many cases are detected before birth or early in life as an incidental finding during evaluations for concerns, such as urinary tract infections [4, 13]. The clinical presentation depends on the age of the patient and the underlying etiology. Neonates are commonly asymptomatic but may present with poor feeding or failure to thrive [14]. Extrinsic UPJO typically manifests during childhood and adolescence and is characterized by symptoms of intermittent mechanical obstruction, such as nausea, vomiting, and flank pain during times of increased diuresis, known as Dietl's Crisis [14, 15]. Other presenting features include recurrent febrile urinary tract infections, hematuria, and nephrolithiasis. Stone crystallization is facilitated by urinary stasis and may be further exacerbated by underlying metabolic abnormalities and impaired passage due to narrowing at the UPJ [5, 16]. Rarely, elevated serum creatinine or new-onset hypertension may prompt investigation and diagnosis of UPJO [17].

Evaluation begins with ultrasonography (**Figure 2**), a non-invasive, first-line imaging modality that effectively demonstrates hydronephrosis. Ultrasonography can measure the degree of renal pelvic dilation, parenchymal thinning, and bladder characteristics, additional factors that may influence the decision to pursue intervention [18]. If UPJO is suspected, functional imaging is performed to evaluate drainage patterns and differential renal function. This is most commonly done with diuretic

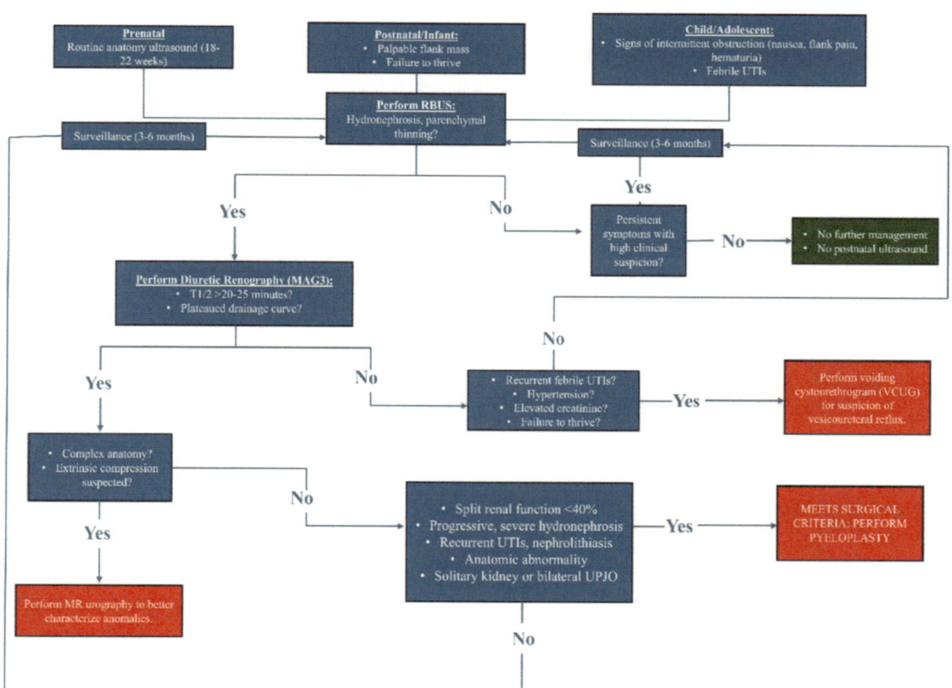

Figure 2.
Flowchart for diagnosis and treatment decisions regarding UPJO.

renography using technetium-99 m mercaptoacetyltriglycine (MAG3), a nuclear medicine study that provides quantifies renal perfusion, function, and excretion [19]. Washout of contrast after administration of a tracer and diuretic, which is rapidly excreted by the kidneys, is assessed. Prolonged half-life of drainage (>20–25 minutes) or a plateaued drainage curve suggests obstruction. A split renal function <40% is also considered significant [11].

Advanced imaging techniques like magnetic resonance urography (MRU) can be valuable for characterizing complex anatomical abnormalities, such as horseshoe kidneys, cross-fused ectopia, or identifying crossed vessels [20]. While voiding cysto-urethrogram (VCUG) is not routinely required, it may be indicated if there is clinical suspicion of concomitant vesicoureteral reflux or lower urinary tract abnormalities [21].

4. Indications for intervention

Not all children diagnosed with UPJO on imaging require surgical correction. Approximately one-third of patients ultimately undergo surgical correction. The decision to proceed with pyeloplasty, the standard surgical treatment, is based on functional imaging, the degree and progression of hydronephrosis, and clinical symptoms [1]. Surgical intervention with pyeloplasty is indicated in the setting of progressive or severe obstruction. One common trigger is declining ipsilateral renal function, with a split renal function (SRF) <40% serving as a threshold for operative management [11]. However, even in patients with stable renal function, progressive worsening of hydronephrosis may warrant surgical evaluation [22]. Other indications include persistent flank pain, recurrent urinary tract infections, obstructive nephrolithiasis, or uncontrolled hypertension attributed to renal obstruction. In rare scenarios such as a solitary kidney or bilateral UPJO, earlier surgical intervention may be warranted given the higher stakes for decline in global renal function [23, 24].

If surgical thresholds are not met, children can be followed closely with serial ultrasounds and repeat diuretic renography [25]. Observation is appropriate when renal function remains stable (greater than 40%), drainage pattern is equivocal or improving, and hydronephrosis is non-progressive. Careful follow-up is essential to detect any deterioration that would necessitate delayed surgical correction. In the case of unilateral UPJO, continuous monitoring of the contralateral kidney for signs of hydronephrosis with ultrasound is necessary.

5. Technique

5.1 Open pyeloplasty

Historically, open dismembered pyeloplasty, as described by Anderson and Hynes, has been the gold standard for surgical correction in both children and adults, boasting long-term success rates exceeding 90% in primary and even reoperative cases [26, 27]. The procedure involves exposing the UPJ through a flank or subcostal incision, excising the obstructed segment, and creating a wide, spatulated, tension-free anastomosis between the renal pelvis and ureter. For infants and young children, modifications such as small, muscle-splitting incisions have proven effective, minimizing morbidity and optimizing cosmetic results, especially beneficial for surgeons who lack robotic experience [26, 28].

The main indications for open pyeloplasty include symptomatic or progressive hydronephrosis, reduced differential renal function (generally less than 40%), recurrent UTIs, renal calculi resulting from obstruction, or pain [6]. In the modern era of prenatal ultrasonography, many cases of hydronephrosis are detected early, and surgery is reserved for those with confirmed obstruction and risk of functional deterioration [26].

The approach is highly versatile, accommodating complex anatomy and prior failed repairs [29]. Complication rates are low; the most common are urinary leak and recurrent stenosis, both generally manageable. Advantages of open pyeloplasty include its proven efficacy, adaptability, and accessibility in all healthcare environments, making it the benchmark for UPJO treatment worldwide [26, 27]. Disadvantages relate to the invasiveness of the technique. Patients typically experience more postoperative pain, longer hospital stays, and have larger or more visible scars compared to minimally invasive approaches. However, minimal-incision and muscle-sparing modifications can lessen these drawbacks, particularly in pediatric patients [28].

The last two decades have witnessed a paradigm shift toward minimally invasive surgical techniques, including conventional laparoscopy and, more recently, robot-assisted approaches. These innovations have been driven by the pursuit of reduced perioperative morbidity, shorter hospital stays, improved cosmesis, and faster recovery, without compromising surgical efficacy.

5.2 Laparoscopic pyeloplasty

Laparoscopic pyeloplasty was first reported in adults in 1993 and soon after in pediatric patients, marking a significant advancement in minimally invasive urologic surgery [30, 31]. The standard technique follows the Anderson-Hynes dismembered technique and may be performed through a transperitoneal or retroperitoneal approach under general anesthesia. In the transperitoneal approach, the patient is placed in a modified flank position; three or four ports are introduced—typically one 5 mm trocar at the umbilicus for the laparoscope and two 3 mm working ports in the upper and lower abdomen, respectively—with the colon mobilized medially to expose the UPJ [24]. The obstructed segment is dissected, excised, and the ureter spatulated before performing a tension-free, watertight ureteropelvic anastomosis using sutures, usually with the insertion of an internal stent for urinary drainage. Retroperitoneoscopic access, less commonly used, involves entering the retroperitoneal space directly, avoiding mobilization of intra-abdominal organs, but offering a more restricted working space [27]. Both transperitoneal and retroperitoneal laparoscopic pyeloplasty have demonstrated high success rates, generally exceeding 90% [32]. Comparative studies suggest that the retroperitoneal approach may offer shorter operative times, reduced hospital stays, and earlier resumption of oral intake, particularly in pediatric populations [33]. However, the retroperitoneal route is technically more demanding due to limited working space and unfamiliar anatomical orientation, contributing to a steeper learning curve and higher conversion rates in some series, particularly early in the learning curve [34]. In adults, both approaches yield comparable functional outcomes, with the choice often dictated by surgeon experience and patient-specific anatomical considerations [35].

Meta-analyses confirm that laparoscopic pyeloplasty achieves success rates similar to open surgery, with the added benefits of reduced postoperative pain, shorter hospital stays, and improved cosmesis [36]. Nevertheless, the technique is technically demanding, requiring advanced laparoscopic skills, particularly for intracorporeal suturing. This limitation has contributed to the gradual shift toward robotic-assisted approaches, especially in centers with access to robotic technology [27].

5.3 Robotic pyeloplasty

Robotic pyeloplasty, first described in 2002, leverages the enhanced dexterity, three-dimensional visualization, and ergonomic advantages of robotic platforms to facilitate complex reconstructive tasks [37]. Robotic pyeloplasty mimics the core steps of the laparoscopic technique but uses three or four robotic ports—a 12 mm camera port, two 8 mm robotic instrument ports, and an optional 5 mm assistant port—most often with a transperitoneal approach (**Figure 3**), although the retroperitoneal route is also feasible [35]. The robot enhances visualization and provides articulating instruments, which greatly facilitate delicate dissection and suturing [27, 38]. Port placement and patient positioning are similar to laparoscopy, but the robotic system allows for more ergonomic and precise movements, potentially reducing operative time and improving surgical outcomes in complex scenarios [38]. The transperitoneal approach remains the most widely adopted for robotic pyeloplasty, offering a broad working field and ease of instrumentation manipulation. However, the retroperitoneal robotic approach is increasingly recognized as feasible and effective, with studies demonstrating comparable operative times, complication rates, and functional outcomes [35, 39]. The retroperitoneal route may be particularly advantageous in patients with prior abdominal surgery or when minimizing peritoneal violation is desired.

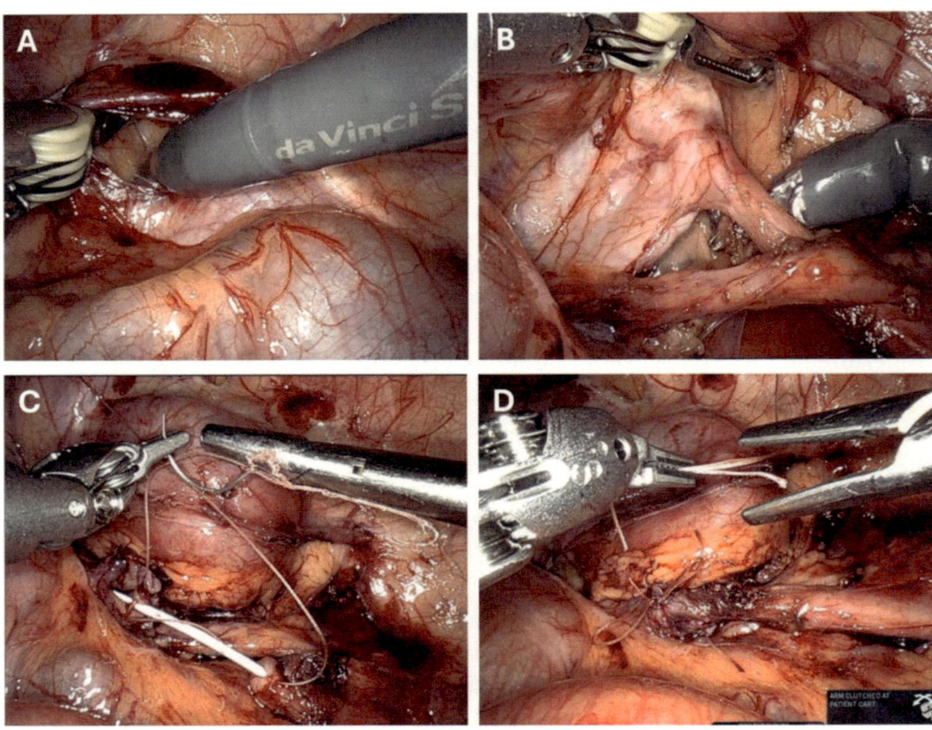

Figure 3.
Robotic pyeloplasty intra-operative images including (A) medial reflection of the colon with exposure of the retroperitoneum, (B) identification of the extrinsic crossing vessel, (C) excision of the atretic segment with (D) reconstruction of the UPJ by re-anastamosing the ureter.

Systematic and meta-analyses indicate that robotic pyeloplasty offers similar success and complication rates to laparoscopic pyeloplasty but with a shorter learning curve, reduced operative times, and lower conversion rates [27, 40]. In both adult and pediatric populations, robotic pyeloplasty is associated with shorter hospital stays and decreased analgesic requirements compared to open surgery [41, 42]. At our high-volume referral center, robotic pyeloplasty is routinely performed using both the Xi and SP platforms. Among two experienced surgeons over the past two years, we have completed over 40 robotic pyeloplasties with a mean length of stay of just 18 hours. Foley catheters are routinely removed on postoperative day one, and patients are discharged the same day, underscoring the feasibility of short-stay or outpatient protocols even in a referral setting. Notably, we have not encountered any postoperative strictures to date. The enhanced precision of robotic suturing is particularly beneficial in complex or redo cases, where tissue planes may be distorted [43]. Robotic pyeloplasty has been shown to be efficacious in children of all body weights [44].

The primary limitations of robotic pyeloplasty are the high cost of robotic systems and limited access in some healthcare settings. Additionally, while the robotic approach reduces the technical demands of intracorporeal suturing, it does not eliminate the need for surgical expertise in reconstructive urology.

5.4 Single-port robotic pyeloplasty

Single-port robotic pyeloplasty represents the latest evolution in minimally invasive UPJO management. The da Vinci SP platform, approved in 2018, allows for the introduction of multiple articulated instruments and a camera through a small single incision, typically 2.5–3.5 cm in length, placed peri-umbilically, mini-Pfannenstiel, or low anterolateral depending on the chosen access [45, 46]. Specialized multi-channel ports are used to introduce a camera and instruments through one site, overcoming instrument clashing with robotically articulated arms in modern systems (**Figure 4**). The surgical steps mirror those of standard pyeloplasty.

Initial series demonstrate that single port robotic pyeloplasty is feasible in both adult and pediatric patients, with operative times, blood loss, and complication rates comparable to multi-port robotic and laparoscopic approaches [45, 47]. Notably, single-port robotic pyeloplasty is associated with shorter hospital stays, reduced

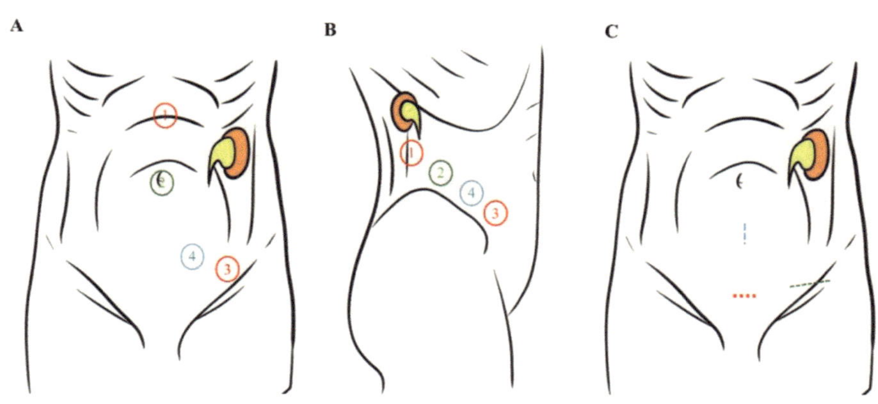

Figure 4.
Port placement for (A) robotic laparoscopic-assisted traditional pyeloplasty and (B) retroperitoneal approach. Green circle is the camera port. Light blue circle is the optional assistant port. (C) Single port approach can be completed with Pfannenstiel (red line), periumbilical (blue line), or low anterolateral (green line).

postoperative pain, and lower opioid requirements, facilitating same-day discharge protocols in select patients [47, 48]. In our practice, same-day discharge is not limited to single-port cases. Even in multi-port robotic pyeloplasty, we discharge patients within 18 hours postoperatively, provided Foley removal on postoperative day 1 is well tolerated and no complications are noted. Cosmetic outcomes are superior due to the single, often hidden incision, which may be particularly relevant in younger or female patients [49].

Meta-analyses comparing single-port to multi-port robotic pyeloplasty reveal no significant differences in operative times, estimated blood loss, complication rates, or success rates [48, 50]. However, single-port robotic pyeloplasty offers advantages in terms of shorter hospital stays, less postoperative pain, and improved cosmetic satisfaction. These benefits are achieved without compromising surgical efficacy or safety, supporting the adoption of single-port robotic pyeloplasty as a viable alternative to traditional multi-port techniques [48].

Single-port robotic pyeloplasty requires specialized equipment and training, and the learning curve, while manageable, may be influenced by prior experience with multi-port robotic surgery. The approach may be limited in patients with high body mass index, extensive prior abdominal surgery, or complex renal anatomy. Long-term data on functional outcomes and durability are still emerging.

5.5 Nephrostomy

Nephrostomy is considered in the management of UPJO primarily when renal function is significantly impaired. Nephrostomy is most often used as a temporary measure in poorly functioning kidneys, especially when SRF is less than 10%, a threshold commonly used to define a non-functioning kidney [51]. Several studies have demonstrated that a period of nephrostomy drainage ranging from 4 to 12 weeks can result in significant improvement in renal function in a substantial proportion of patients. For instance, a pediatric cohort reported that the mean SRF improved from 6.67% to 16.80% after three months of nephrostomy, with corresponding increases in effective renal plasma flow [51]. All patients in this series subsequently underwent successful pyeloplasty, obviating the need for nephrectomy. Similarly, 56.6% of adult patients with initial SRF <10% demonstrated functional improvement after nephrostomy, particularly among younger adults, thus qualifying them for reconstructive surgery rather than nephrectomy [52].

In addition to its role in preoperative assessment, nephrostomy may be employed as a protective measure following pyeloplasty, particularly in complex or high-risk cases. Nephrostomy tube drainage can help prevent urinary extravasation, facilitate radiographic assessment of anastomosis, and provide access for further intervention if needed [53]. Large series have demonstrated that nephrostomy tube drainage after pyeloplasty is associated with low complication rates and does not prolong hospitalization, making it a reasonable option in selected patients [53].

5.6 Nephrectomy

Nephrectomy, the surgical removal of the affected kidney, is generally considered when the likelihood of functional recovery is minimal or when the kidney poses a risk to the patient's health. A Dimercaptosuccinic acid (DMSA) scan should be obtained to confirm clinical suspicion. While MAG-3 is used to assess renal perfusion, function, and drainage, DMSA is primarily used for static renal cortical imaging. DMSA is highly effective in detecting focal parenchymal abnormalities, such as scarring, and provides reliable assessment of differential renal function. Traditional indications for nephrectomy in the context of UPJO include persistently low SRF of less than 10% after a period of urinary diversion. For example, if a nephrostomy does not result in meaningful improvement in renal function or urine output remains low (<400 ml/day), nephrectomy is warranted [52]. Additionally, recurrent or refractory symptoms such as persistent pain, infection, or hypertension attributable to the non-functioning kidney may necessitate nephrectomy, particularly when these symptoms are not controlled by conservative or reconstructive measures [54, 55]. Shared decision making should be employed to inform patients entirely.

6. Challenging cases

6.1 Recurrent UPJO

Recurrent UPJO following initial pyeloplasty is a significant surgical challenge, often necessitating reoperative intervention. The etiology of recurrence may include technical failure, ischemia, or missed crossing vessels, and the presence of fibrosis and adhesions complicates subsequent repairs [38]. Redo pyeloplasty, particularly performed robotically, has demonstrated high success rates, with reported outcomes ranging from 78 to 100% in pediatric series [38]. The robotic approach offers enhanced visualization and dexterity, facilitating meticulous dissection in scarred fields and allowing for anterior approaches that may avoid previously operated tissue planes. In select cases where reconstruction is not feasible due to extensive scarring, robotic ureterocalycostomy has been described as a viable alternative. In our institutional experience managing referred redo pyeloplasties, we favor generous ureteral spatulation and tension-free anastomosis, reinforced with biologic adjuncts such as AmnioFix. We also recapitulate the retroperitoneum and avoid routine drain placement. These technical strategies, paried with the robotic platform's enhanced precision, have contributed to consistent success in challenging reoperative settings.

Endopyelotomy, either antegrade or retrograde, has also been utilized in the management of recurrent UPJO. While technically less invasive, its success rates are generally inferior to those of redo pyeloplasty. In a retrospective review, secondary pyeloplasty achieved an overall success rate of 87.5%, compared to 44% for secondary endopyelotomy [56]. Long-term follow-up studies have reported sustained success rates of 87.5% for endopyelotomy after failed pyeloplasty, but outcomes are significantly worse in the presence of poor renal function or severe hydronephrosis [57]. Thus, while endopyelotomy may be considered in select adult patients with favorable anatomy and preserved renal function, redo pyeloplasty remains the preferred approach in most pediatric and complex cases.

6.2 Anatomic variants

Anatomic variants such as horseshoe kidney, pelvic kidney, malrotated kidney, and duplex systems introduce additional complexity to pyeloplasty. Aberrant vasculature, abnormal renal rotation, and altered relationships between the renal pelvis and ureter can complicate both exposure and reconstruction [58]. Robotic-assisted laparoscopic pyeloplasty has been shown to be feasible and effective in these scenarios, with the advantages of three-dimensional visualization and precise instrument control aiding in the identification and preservation of aberrant vessels [58]. In a multicenter review, robotic-assisted laparoscopic pyeloplasty was successfully completed in cases involving horseshoe kidney, pelvic kidneys, and duplex systems, with no conversions to open surgery and 95% overall success rate at three years [58].

6.3 Poorly functioning kidneys

The management of UPJO in poorly functioning kidneys—typically defined as SRF less than 20–30%—remains controversial. Historically, nephrectomy was often favored due to concerns regarding the potential for functional recovery and the risk of persistent symptoms or complications including chronic infection or recurrent nephrolithiasis [59]. However, recent evidence suggests that pyeloplasty can result in stabilization or even improvement of renal function in a substantial proportion of these patients [60, 61]. In a large series, pyeloplasty in adults with SRF $\leq$ 20% achieved functional success in 95.6% of cases, with significant improvements in SRF and drainage parameters at long-term follow-up [60]. Similar findings have been reported in pediatric populations, with functional recovery observed in up to one-third of children and stable function in the majority of the remainder [61].

6.4 Infants and low-weight children

Infants and low-weight children (<6 kg) present unique technical and physiological challenges for pyeloplasty. The small working space, delicate tissues, and increased risk of anesthesia-related complications necessitate meticulous surgical planning and execution [38, 58]. Robotic-assisted pyeloplasty has been successfully performed in infants, with outcomes comparable to open surgery and the added benefits of reduced postoperative pain and shorter hospital stays [38, 44, 62, 63]. In a multicenter review, robotic-assisted laparoscopic pyeloplasty was completed without conversion in 10 infants weighing less than 6 kg, with a 95% success rate and minimal complications [58].

Endopyelotomy is generally not recommended in infants and young children due to poor outcomes and higher failure rates [64]. In a limited series, 75% of endopyelotomies in children under five years failed, underscoring the need for formal reconstructive surgery in this population [64].

6.5 The use of endopyelotomy

Endopyelotomy involves the endoscopic incision of the UPJO, typically performed through an antegrade percutaneous or retrograde ureteroscopic approach. The procedure may utilize a cold knife, electrocautery, or laser, and is often followed by stent placement to maintain patency during healing. Indications for endopyelotomy include both primary UPJO and secondary cases, such as recurrent obstruction after failed pyeloplasty or iatrogenic strictures following renal surgery [64]. Patient selection is critical when considering endopyelotomy. This procedure is typically reserved for patients who do not have significant crossing vessels, have relatively preserved preoperative renal function, lack severe hydronephrosis, and are not young children [57, 65, 66].

Short-term success of endopyelotomy is typically defined by symptomatic relief and radiographic evidence of unobstructed drainage within the first 6–12 months post-procedure. Reported short-term success rates for endopyelotomy in primary UPJO are nearly 90% [66, 67]. For secondary UPJO, success rates are similar, with some series reporting up to 83.5% after failed pyeloplasty [64].

Long-term follow-up is essential to accurately assess the durability of endopyelotomy. Several studies have demonstrated a decline in success rates over time. For example, DiMarco et al. reported 3-, 5-, and 10- year recurrence-free survival rates of 63%, 55%, and 41%, respectively, for endopyelotomy, compared to 85%, 80%, and 75% for pyeloplasty [68]. Similarly, Doo et al. found that success rates decreased from 87.8% at 6 months to 61.6% at 60 months [67]. These findings underscore the importance of extended follow-up, as late failures can occur even several years post-procedure. Despite this decline, endopyelotomy remains a valuable option, particularly for select patient populations. In the context of secondary UPJO, long-term success rates remain favorable, with Jabbour et al. reporting an 87.5% sustained success rate after a mean follow-up of 88.5 months [57]. Vaarala et al. also demonstrated durable results, with 94% of patients experiencing improved radiographic outcomes and 100% patient satisfaction after antegrade endopyelotomy, with a mean follow-up of over 12 years [69].

7. Management of complications

Complications such as anastomotic urine leak and obstruction following pyeloplasty, while infrequent, remain clinically significant. Historically, conservative approaches such as prolonged surgical drainage, urethral catheterization, and observation have been employed, particularly for urine leaks [70]. While some cases resolve spontaneously, persistent leakage or obstruction may necessitate more aggressive intervention to prevent fibrosis and loss of function. Emerging evidence supports the early use of percutaneous nephrostomy as an effective intervention for both anastomotic leaks and acute obstruction after pyeloplasty [71]. The rationale for prompt nephrostomy placement is twofold—it provides effective urinary diversion, thereby minimizing peri-anastomotic urine exposure and the risk of fibrosis, and it avoids premature stent manipulation, which could compromise anastomotic healing. Furthermore, nephrostomy allows for antegrade assessment of the anastomosis and timely intervention should persistent obstruction be identified. In cases where poor drainage persists despite initial management, percutaneous balloon dilation of the anastomosis can be considered, typically after a 4–6 week period to allow for resolution of postoperative edema and adequate tissue healing [59]. For patients with recurrent or persistent obstruction after initial pyeloplasty, secondary interventions include redo pyeloplasty, endopyelotomy, or, in select cases, nephrectomy. Evidence consistently demonstrates superior outcomes for redo pyeloplasty compared to endopyelotomy [56]. Endopyelotomy may be considered in select patients, particularly those unfit for major surgery, but is associated with lower long-term success.

8. Conclusion

Pyeloplasty stands as the definitive treatment for UPJO, achieving consistently high rates of long-term success in both pediatric and adult populations. The landscape of UPJO management has been transformed by advancements in imaging and surgical technology, allowing for earlier diagnosis, accurate assessment of renal function, and minimally invasive surgical options that enhance patient recovery and satisfaction. Laparoscopic and robotic-assisted techniques have largely replaced open surgery, offering comparable effectiveness with the added benefits of reduced pain, shorter hospitalization, and superior cosmetic outcomes. Management strategies must be tailored to individual patient factors, such as age, anatomy, renal function, and the presence of complex or recurrent disease, to ensure optimal outcomes. Special populations, including infants, patients with anatomic variants, or those with severely impaired renal function, require nuanced approaches and multidisciplinary expertise. Adjunct procedures, including nephrostomy and nephrectomy, retain important roles in select clinical scenarios. As the field continues to evolve, ongoing research and technological innovation promise further refinements in the diagnosis and management of UPJO. Through a combination of evidence-based practice, personalized patient care, and technical advances, clinicians are increasingly able to preserve renal function, reduce morbidity, and improve the quality of life for individuals affected by this condition.

Acknowledgements

The authors declare no funding for this original book chapter.

Conflict of interest

The authors declare no conflict of interest.

Author details

Jason Yang, Aidan Weitzner and Chad Crigger*
Robert D. Jeffs Division of Pediatric Urology, James Buchanan Brady Urological Institutions, Johns Hopkins Hospital, Johns Hopkins Medical Institutions, Charlotte Bloomberg Children's Hospital, Baltimore, MD, USA

*Address all correspondence to: ccrigge2@jh.edu

References

[1] Fwu CW, Barthold JS, Mendley SR, et al. Epidemiology of infantile ureteropelvic junction obstruction in the US. Urology. 2024;**183**:185-191. DOI: 10.1016/j.urology.2023.09.024

[2] Roth CC, Hubanks JM, Bright BC, et al. Occurrence of urinary tract infection in children with significant upper urinary tract obstruction. Urology. 2009;**73**(1):74-78. DOI: 10.1016/j.urology.2008.05.021

[3] Alberti C. Congenital ureteropelvic junction obstruction: Physiopathology, decoupling of tout court pelvic dilatation-obstruction semantic connection, biomarkers to predict renal damage evolution. European Review for Medical and Pharmacological Sciences. 2012;**16**(2):213-219

[4] Krajewski W, Wojciechowska J, Dembowski J, Zdrojowy R, Szydełko T. Hydronephrosis in the course of ureteropelvic junction obstruction: An underestimated problem? Current opinions on the pathogenesis, diagnosis and treatment. Advances in Clinical and Experimental Medicine: Official Organ Wroclaw Medical University. 2017;**26**(5):857-864. DOI: 10.17219/acem/59509

[5] Leavitt DA, de la Rosette JJMCH, Hoenig DM. Strategies for nonmedical management of upper urinary tract calculi. In: Partin AW, Peters CA, Kavoussi LR, Dmochowski RR, Wein AJ, editors. Campbell-Walsh-Wein Urology. 12th ed. Pennsylvania: Elsevier; 2020. pp. 2069-2093

[6] González R, Schimke CM. Ureteropelvic junction obstruction in infants and children. Pediatric Clinics of North America. 2001;**48**(6):1505-1518. DOI: 10.1016/s0031-3955(05)70388-6

[7] Kim JK, Keefe DT, Rickard M, Milford K, Lorenzo AJ, Chua ME. Vascular hitch for paediatric pelvi-ureteric junction obstruction with crossing vessels: Institutional analysis and systematic review with meta-analysis. BJU International. 2022;**129**(6):679-687. DOI: 10.1111/bju.15342

[8] Mitterberger M, Pinggera GM, Neururer R, et al. Comparison of contrast-enhanced color Doppler imaging (CDI), computed tomography (CT), and magnetic resonance imaging (MRI) for the detection of crossing vessels in patients with ureteropelvic junction obstruction (UPJO). European Urology. 2008;**53**(6):1254-1262. DOI: 10.1016/j.eururo.2007.11.031

[9] Herthelius M. Antenatally detected urinary tract dilatation: Long-term outcome. Pediatric Nephrology. 2023;**38**(10):3221-3227. DOI: 10.1007/s00467-023-05907-z

[10] Lim DJ, Park JY, Kim JH, Paick SH, Oh SJ, Choi H. Clinical characteristics and outcome of hydronephrosis detected by prenatal ultrasonography. Journal of Korean Medical Science. 2003;**18**(6):859. DOI: 10.3346/jkms.2003.18.6.859

[11] Gordon I, Dhillon HK, Gatanash H, Peters AM. Antenatal diagnosis of pelvic hydronephrosis: Assessment of renal function and drainage as a guide to management. Journal of Nuclear Medicine: Official of Society of Nuclear Medicine. 1991;**32**(9):1649-1654

[12] Joan Robson W, Rudy SM, Johnston JH. Pelviureteric obstruction in infancy. Journal of Pediatric

Surgery. 1976;**11**(1):57-61. DOI: 10.1016/0022-3468(76)90170-6

[13] Has R, Sarac ST. Prenatal diagnosis and findings in ureteropelvic junction type hydronephrosis. Frontiers in Pediatrics. 2020;**8**:492. DOI: 10.3389/fped.2020.00492

[14] El-Dahr SS, Lewy JE. Urinary tract obstruction and infection in the neonate. Clinics in Perinatology. 1992;**19**(1):213-222

[15] Flotte TR. Dietl syndrome: Intermittent ureteropelvic junction obstruction as a cause of episodic abdominal pain. Pediatrics. 1988;**82**(5):792-794. DOI: 10.1542/peds.82.5.792

[16] Tekin A, Tekgul S, Atsu N, Ergen A, Kendi S. Ureteropelvic junction obstruction and coexisting renal calculi in children: Role of metabolic abnormalities. Urology. 2001;**57**(3):542-545. DOI: 10.1016/S0090-4295(00)01030-X

[17] Chandrasekharam V, Shah M, Padua M, Babu R, Vittalraj P, Sundaram S. Results of temporary drainage of poorly functioning kidneys with ureteropelvic junction obstruction: Does the histology of persistent poor functioning kidneys indicate an increased risk of hypertension? Urology. 2024;**184**:189-194. DOI: 10.1016/j.urology.2023.10.011

[18] Dias CS, Silva JMP, Pereira AK, et al. Diagnostic accuracy of renal pelvic dilatation for detecting surgically managed ureteropelvic junction obstruction. The Journal of Urology. 2013;**190**(2):661-666. DOI: 10.1016/j.juro.2013.02.014

[19] Majd M, Bar-Sever Z, Santos AI, De Palma D. The SNMMI and EANM procedural guidelines for diuresis renography in infants and children. Journal of Nuclear Medicine. 2018;**59**(10):1636-1640. DOI: 10.2967/jnumed.118.215921

[20] Parikh KR, Hammer MR, Kraft KH, Ivančić V, Smith EA, Dillman JR. Pediatric ureteropelvic junction obstruction: Can magnetic resonance urography identify crossing vessels? Pediatric Radiology. 2015;**45**(12):1788-1795. DOI: 10.1007/s00247-015-3412-y

[21] Hubertus J, Plieninger S, Martinovic V, et al. Children and adolescents with ureteropelvic junction obstruction: Is an additional voiding cystourethrogram necessary? Results of a multicenter study. World Journal of Urology. 2013;**31**(3):683-687. DOI: 10.1007/s00345-012-0918-x

[22] Chertin B, Pollack A, Koulikov D, et al. Conservative treatment of ureteropelvic junction obstruction in children with antenatal diagnosis of hydronephrosis: Lessons learned after 16 years of follow-up. European Urology. 2006;**49**(4):734-739. DOI: 10.1016/j.eururo.2006.01.046

[23] Cai PY, Lee RS. Ureteropelvic junction obstruction/hydronephrosis. The Urologic Clinics of North America. 2023;**50**(3):361-369. DOI: 10.1016/j.ucl.2023.04.001

[24] Szavay P. Laparoscopic pyeloplasty for ureteropelvic junction obstruction. Journal of Laparoendoscopic & Advanced Surgical Techniques. Part A. 2021;**31**(10):1214-1218. DOI: 10.1089/lap.2021.0452

[25] Heinlen JE, Manatt CS, Bright BC, Kropp BP, Campbell JB, Frimberger D. Operative versus nonoperative management of ureteropelvic junction

obstruction in children. Urology. 2009;**73**(3):521-525. DOI: 10.1016/j.urology.2008.08.512

[26] Sutherland RW, Chung SK, Roth DR, Gonzales ET. Pediatric pyeloplasty: Outcome analysis based on patient age and surgical technique. Urology. 1997;**50**(6):963-966. DOI: 10.1016/S0090-4295(97)00397-X

[27] Autorino R, Eden C, El-Ghoneimi A, et al. Robot-assisted and laparoscopic repair of ureteropelvic junction obstruction: A systematic review and meta-analysis. European Urology. 2014;**65**(2):430-452. DOI: 10.1016/j.eururo.2013.06.053

[28] Chacko JK, Koyle MA, Mingin GC, Furness PD 3rd. The minimally invasive open pyeloplasty. Journal of Pediatric Urology. 2006;**2**(4):368-372. DOI: 10.1016/j.jpurol.2006.05.001

[29] Thomas JC, DeMarco RT, Donohoe JM, Adams MC, Pope JC 4th, Brock JW 3rd. Management of the failed pyeloplasty: A contemporary review. The Journal of Urology. 2005;**174**(6):2363-2366. DOI: 10.1097/01.ju.0000180420.11915.31

[30] Peters CA, Schlussel RN, Retik AB. Pediatric laparoscopic dismembered pyeloplasty. The Journal of Urology. 1995;**153**(6):1962-1965

[31] Schuessler WW, Grune MT, Tecuanhuey LV, Preminger GM. Laparoscopic dismembered pyeloplasty. The Journal of Urology. 1993;**150**(6):1795-1799. DOI: 10.1016/s0022-5347(17)35898-6

[32] Rassweiler JJ, Teber D, Frede T. Complications of laparoscopic pyeloplasty. World Journal of Urology. 2008;**26**(6):539-547. DOI: 10.1007/s00345-008-0266-z

[33] Badawy H, Zoaier A, Ghoneim T, Hanno A. Transperitoneal versus retroperitoneal laparoscopic pyeloplasty in children: Randomized clinical trial. Journal of Pediatric Urology. 2015;**11**(3):122.e1-122.e6. DOI: 10.1016/j.jpurol.2014.11.019

[34] Wu Y, Dong Q, Han P, Liu L, Wang L, Wei Q. Meta-analysis of transperitoneal versus retroperitoneal approaches of laparoscopic pyeloplasty for ureteropelvic junction obstruction. Journal of Laparoendoscopic & Advanced Surgical Techniques. Part A. 2012;**22**(7):658-662. DOI: 10.1089/lap.2011.0508

[35] Cestari A, Buffi NM, Lista G, et al. Retroperitoneal and transperitoneal robot-assisted pyeloplasty in adults: Techniques and results. European Urology. 2010;**58**(5):711-718. DOI: 10.1016/j.eururo.2010.07.020

[36] Mei H, Pu J, Yang C, Zhang H, Zheng L, Tong Q. Laparoscopic versus open pyeloplasty for ureteropelvic junction obstruction in children: A systematic review and meta-analysis. Journal of Endourology. 2011;**25**(5):727-736. DOI: 10.1089/end.2010.0544

[37] Gettman MT, Neururer R, Bartsch G, Peschel R. Anderson-Hynes dismembered pyeloplasty performed using the da Vinci robotic system. Urology. 2002;**60**(3):509-513. DOI: 10.1016/S0090-4295(02)01761-2

[38] Boysen WR, Gundeti MS. Robot-assisted laparoscopic pyeloplasty in the pediatric population: A review of technique, outcomes, complications, and special considerations in infants. Pediatric Surgery International. 2017;**33**(9):925-935. DOI: 10.1007/s00383-017-4082-7

[39] Kaouk JH, Hafron J, Parekattil S, et al. Is retroperitoneal approach feasible

for robotic dismembered pyeloplasty: Initial experience and long-term results. Journal of Endourology. 2008;**22**(9):2153-2159. DOI: 10.1089/end.2008.0130

[40] Braga LHP, Pace K, DeMaria J, Lorenzo AJ. Systematic review and meta-analysis of robotic-assisted versus conventional laparoscopic pyeloplasty for patients with ureteropelvic junction obstruction: Effect on operative time, length of hospital stay, postoperative complications, and success rate. European Urology. 2009;**56**(5):848-857. DOI: 10.1016/j.eururo.2009.03.063

[41] Yee DS, Shanberg AM, Duel BP, Rodriguez E, Eichel L, Rajpoot D. Initial comparison of robotic-assisted laparoscopic versus open pyeloplasty in children. Urology. 2006;**67**(3):599-602. DOI: 10.1016/j.urology.2005.09.021

[42] Lee RS, Retik AB, Borer JG, Peters CA. Pediatric robot assisted laparoscopic dismembered pyeloplasty: Comparison with a cohort of open surgery. The Journal of Urology. 2006;**175**(2):683-687; discussion 687. DOI: 10.1016/S0022-5347(05)00183-7

[43] Lindgren BW, Hagerty J, Meyer T, Cheng EY. Robot-assisted laparoscopic reoperative repair for failed pyeloplasty in children: A safe and highly effective treatment option. The Journal of Urology. 2012;**188**(3):932-937. DOI: 10.1016/j.juro.2012.04.118

[44] Masieri L, Sforza S, Grosso AA, et al. Does the body weight influence the outcome in children treated with robotic pyeloplasty? Journal of Pediatric Urology. 2020;**16**(1):109.e1-109.e6. DOI: 10.1016/j.jpurol.2019.10.023

[45] Ramos R, Chavali JS, Ferguson E, et al. Low anterolateral incision for single-port extraperitoneal robot-assisted pyeloplasty: Description of technique and initial experience. World Journal of Urology. 2024;**42**(1):263. DOI: 10.1007/s00345-024-04915-4

[46] Lenfant L, Wilson CA, Sawczyn G, Aminsharifi A, Kim S, Kaouk J. Single-port robot-assisted dismembered pyeloplasty with mini-pfannenstiel or peri-umbilical access: Initial experience in a single center. Urology. 2020;**143**:147-152. DOI: 10.1016/j.urology.2020.05.041

[47] Beksac AT, Wilson CA, Lenfant L, et al. Single-port mini-pfannenstiel robotic pyeloplasty: Establishing a non-narcotic pathway along with a same-day discharge protocol. Urology. 2022;**160**:130-135. DOI: 10.1016/j.urology.2021.10.013

[48] Gu L, Li Y, Li X, Liu W. Single-port vs multiple-port robot-assisted laparoscopic pyeloplasty for the treatment of ureteropelvic junction obstruction: A systematic review and meta-analysis. Journal of Endourology. 2023;**37**(6):681-687. DOI: 10.1089/end.2023.0064

[49] Gargollo PC. Hidden incision endoscopic surgery: Description of technique, parental satisfaction and applications. The Journal of Urology. 2011;**185**(4):1425-1431. DOI: 10.1016/j.juro.2010.11.054

[50] Harrison J, Maguire P, Pitceathly C. Confiding in crisis: Gender differences in pattern of confiding among cancer patients. Social Science & Medicine. 1995;**41**(9):1255-1260. DOI: 10.1016/0277-9536(94)00411-L

[51] Rai RK, Pandey A, Verma S, et al. Management of non-functioning kidney due to pelvi-ureteric junction obstruction in pediatric age group: An observational study. Pediatric Surgery

International. 2023;**39**(1):85. DOI: 10.1007/s00383-023-05368-3

[52] Zhang S, Zhang Q, Ji C, et al. Improved split renal function after percutaneous nephrostomy in young adults with severe hydronephrosis due to ureteropelvic junction obstruction. The Journal of Urology. 2015;**193**(1):191-195. DOI: 10.1016/j.juro.2014.07.005

[53] Austin PF, Cain MP, Rink RC. Nephrostomy tube drainage with pyeloplasty: Is it necessarily a bad choice? The Journal of Urology. 2000;**163**(5):1528-1530. DOI: 10.1016/s0022-5347(05)67671-9

[54] Hemal AK, Mishra S. Retroperitoneoscopic nephrectomy for pyonephrotic nonfunctioning kidney. Urology. 2010;**75**(3):585-588. DOI: 10.1016/j.urology.2008.07.054

[55] Elhage O, Sahai A, Challacombe B, Murphy D, Scoble J, Dasgupta P. Role of laparoscopic nephrectomy for refractory hypertension in poorly functioning kidneys. Annals of the Royal College of Surgeons of England. 2011;**93**(1):25-26. DOI: 10.1308/003588410X12771863936800

[56] Vannahme M, Mathur S, Davenport K, Timoney AG, Keeley FX. The management of secondary pelvi-ureteric junction obstruction - a comparison of pyeloplasty and endopyelotomy. BJU International. 2014;**113**(1):108-112. DOI: 10.1111/bju.12454

[57] Jabbour ME, Goldfischer ER, Klima WJ, Stravodimos KG, Smith AD. Endopyelotomy after failed pyeloplasty: The long-term results. The Journal of Urology. 1998;**160**(3 Pt 1):690-692; discussion 692-693. DOI: 10.1016/S0022-5347(01)62757-5

[58] Chertin L, Verhovsky G, Jaber J, et al. Robotic-assisted laparoscopic pyeloplasty in challenging cases of ureteropelvic junction obstruction in the pediatric population: A multicenter review. Journal of Laparoendoscopic & Advanced Surgical Techniques. Part A. 2024;**34**(5):443-447. DOI: 10.1089/lap.2023.0205

[59] Miyamoto KK, Mesrobian HG. Long-term outcome of kidneys with initially poor drainage or no drainage following pyeloplasty. World Journal of Urology. 1996;**14**(6):380-383. DOI: 10.1007/BF00183119

[60] Elbaset MA, Zahran MH, Sharaf MA, et al. Long term functional success after pyeloplasty for pelvi-ureteral junction obstruction in unilateral poorly functioning kidney in exclusively adults population. Urology. 2019;**131**:234-239. DOI: 10.1016/j.urology.2019.05.030

[61] Sarhan O, Al Otay A, Al Faddagh A, et al. Pyeloplasty in children with low differential renal function: Functional recoverability. Journal of Pediatric Urology. 2021;**17**(5):658.e1-658.e9. DOI: 10.1016/j.jpurol.2021.07.003

[62] Reed F, Recabal X, Echeverría P, et al. Are weight or age limits for pediatric laparoscopic pyeloplasty? Results of a multicentric study. World Journal of Urology. 2023;**41**(6):1675-1679. DOI: 10.1007/s00345-023-04359-2

[63] Andolfi C, Rodríguez VM, Galansky L, Gundeti MS. Infant robot-assisted laparoscopic pyeloplasty: Outcomes at a single institution, and tips for safety and success. European Urology. 2021;**80**(5):621-631. DOI: 10.1016/j.eururo.2021.06.019

[64] Patel T, Kellner CP, Katsumi H, Gupta M. Efficacy of endopyelotomy in

patients with secondary ureteropelvic junction obstruction. Journal of Endourology. 2011;**25**(4):587-591. DOI: 10.1089/end.2010.0026

[65] Knudsen BE, Cook AJ, Watterson JD, et al. Percutaneous antegrade endopyelotomy: Long-term results from one institution. Urology. 2004;**63**(2):230-234. DOI: 10.1016/j.urology.2003.09.049

[66] Danuser H, Ackermann DK, Böhlen D, Studer UE. Endopyelotomy for primary ureteropelvic junction obstruction: Risk factors determine the success rate. The Journal of Urology. 1998;**159**(1):56-61. DOI: 10.1016/s0022-5347(01)64011-4

[67] Doo CK, Hong B, Park T, Park HK. Long-term outcome of endopyelotomy for the treatment of ureteropelvic junction obstruction: How long should patients be followed up? Journal of Endourology. 2007;**21**(2):158-161. DOI: 10.1089/end.2006.0191

[68] Dimarco DS, Gettman MT, McGee SM, et al. Long-term success of antegrade endopyelotomy compared with pyeloplasty at a single institution. Journal of Endourology. 2006;**20**(10):707-712. DOI: 10.1089/end.2006.20.707

[69] Vaarala MH, Marttila T, Paananen I, Hellström P. Retrospective analysis of long-term outcomes of 64 patients treated by endopyelotomy in two low-volume hospitals: Good and durable results. Journal of Endourology. 2008;**22**(8):1659-1664. DOI: 10.1089/end.2008.0117

[70] Wolf JS. Laparoscopic transperitoneal pyeloplasty. Journal of Endourology. 2011;**25**(2):173-178. DOI: 10.1089/end.2010.0605

[71] Ozayar A, Morgan MSC, Friedlander JI, et al. Prompt management of anastomotic leak or acute obstruction after minimally invasive pyeloplasty with percutaneous nephrostomy preserves outcomes. The Journal of Urology. 2014;**192**(6):1716-1719. DOI: 10.1016/j.juro.2014.06.041

Section 4

Pediatric Functional Surgery

Chapter 7

Advances in Pediatric Epilepsy Surgery

Ryan Kelly, Melissa A. LoPresti and Sandi Lam

Abstract

Epilepsy effects over 50 million people worldwide. Of those, 20–40% of children with epilepsy are considered medically refractory. When pharmacotherapy fails, surgical intervention remains an option to achieve seizure freedom or reduce seizure burden. In this chapter, we review the relevant presurgical evaluation patients undergo, the role of invasive monitoring, and the various types of epilepsy surgery that may help treat children with refractory epilepsy. We discuss in detail various types of surgery, including conventional resection, lobectomy, and disconnection surgeries, as well as innovations in the field including neuromodulation and LITT. We provide a comprehensive review of the current status of the field and highlight future directions.

Keywords: epilepsy, refractory epilepsy, epilepsy surgery, neuromodulation, pediatric neurosurgery

1. Introduction

Epilepsy is a heterogeneous neurological condition hallmarked by recurrent seizures affecting either part of or the whole body with or without impaired consciousness. It is thought that over 50 million people around the world live with epilepsy, with a cumulative incidence of 67.77 per 100,000 persons [1]. It has long been recognized that epilepsy affects pediatric patients at greater rates compared to their adult counterparts, with an estimated 10.5 million children affected worldwide with incidences of 85.29 per 100,000 persons in patients under 18 years of age, compared to 64.81 per 100,000 persons in patients over 19 years of age [1, 2]. In a separate study, it was found that the incidence of pediatric epilepsy was highest during the first year of life at 144 per 100,000 persons and decreases throughout the first decade [3].

It is imperative that pediatric patients with frequent seizures achieve disease freedom as continued epileptogenic activity can cause regression of or arrest cerebral maturation, possibly delaying cognitive development [4, 5]. In addition, mortality in those living with continued seizure is higher than those in age-matched populations [6–9]. In order to reduce the frequency and intensity of seizures, patients are placed on various antiseizure medications (ASM) that alter neurotransmitter action and electrical propagation throughout the brain. These medications can be associated with varying adverse effects with some patients being placed on multiple medications despite poor seizure control. Regardless of medications, approximately 20–40%

IntechOpen

of pediatric patients will develop drug-resistant epilepsy (DRE), which represents persistent seizures despite adequate trials of at least two different ASMs [10]. Patients with this pharmaco-resistant form of epilepsy are more susceptible to cognitive problems, mood and personality changes, educational and social consequences, persistent seizures, increased risk of mortality, and comorbidities that greatly reduce the patient's and family's quality of life [11, 12]. In a study defining long-term survival of pediatric patients with drug-resistant epilepsy by treatment type, those with cranial epilepsy surgery had a 98% chance of being alive at 10 years, while those with vagus nerve stimulation had a 92% chance of being alive at 10 years, and those on medical treatment only had an 89% chance of being alive at 10 years [13].

When pharmacotherapy fails, surgical intervention is recommended to achieve seizure freedom or reduce seizure burden. Traditionally centered on open surgery, either for resection of the epileptogenic focus or disconnection of neural pathways involved in epilepsy networks, epilepsy surgery has grown significantly since its inception to include neuromodulation and more minimally invasive approaches [9, 14]. In this chapter, we discuss the evolution of epilepsy surgery over time, focusing on the traditional approaches as well as current advances in the field of pediatric epilepsy surgery.

With the development of improved pharmaceutical options and more advanced operative techniques, the indications for epilepsy surgery has evolved over the past several decades. In 2009, the International League Against Epilepsy (ILAE) defined DRE and recommended surgical resection, if possible [15]. Additional conditions that can benefit from surgical intervention include certain pathologies such as cortical dysplasia, Sturge–Weber Syndrome, Rasmussen syndrome, and/or seizure semiology that can be localized to a specific location or lesion [16, 17]. While the role of surgery has expanded to include those with nonlesional epilepsy, some patients such as those with active psychiatric illnesses, severe medical co-morbidities, or no discernable epileptogenic focus or network are less likely to benefit from surgical treatment [16]. Jehi et al. in an international panel and modified Delphi methodology presented expert consensus defining recommendations for timely referral of patients who could benefit from evaluation for epilepsy surgery, which included: (1) every patient <70 years of age as soon as they meet criteria for drug-resistant epilepsy; (2) patients >70 years of age with drug-resistant epilepsy with no surgical contraindication; (3) patients of any age who are seizure-free on 1–2 antiseizure medications with a brain lesion in non-eloquent cortex. Jehi et al. recommended against referral for epilepsy surgery for those with active substance abuse problems not cooperative with management [18]. In appropriately selected patients who undergo epilepsy surgery, long-term seizure control rates can range from 50 to 70% [19]. However, despite improved patient selection and operative techniques, surgical intervention remains underutilized with approximately 1% of the 100,000–500,000 eligible patients undergoing surgery annually [20].

2. Presurgical evaluation and workup

The goal of surgery is to minimize damaging effects of epilepsy on the developing brain caused by recurrent seizures and antiseizure medications. This is increasingly important in children due to the neuroplasticity of the young, developing brain and the need to prevent damage and allow proper development to occur. While surgery has become an invaluable resource for many patients with DRE, there are a number of significant steps that must be undertaken by the patient and healthcare providers prior to intervention.

2.1 Phase I evaluation

The typical workup for epilepsy can be divided into several stepwise phases to ensure optimal patient selection and treatment modality. Phase I consists of understanding the seizure semiology and obtaining neuroimaging to look for pathologic areas that might correlate with seizure focus (**Table 1**). All initial evaluations should begin with a detailed clinical history to determine the semiology, triggers, and frequency of seizures as well as a physical exam to evaluate for neurological deficits or abnormalities. Intracranial imaging with a magnetic resonance imaging (MRI) should be completed to rule out any structural etiology (i.e. hippocampal sclerosis, neoplasm, or cortical dysplasia) as the source of the patient's seizures. The next step in the work-up is to characterize the seizure using an interictal scalp electroencephalography (EEG) via long-term video monitoring. Patients should be evaluated by neuropsychology/neuropsychiatry to determine any subtle neurological deficits as well as baseline cognitive ability and reserve. Additional testing with magnetoencephalogram (MEG) and functional MRI (fMRI) can be used to localize eloquent cortical structures while interictal positron emission tomography (PET) and ictal photon emission computed tomography can demonstrate hypometabolism and increased cerebral blood flow within the epileptic foci helping to better localize it [10].

2.2 Phase II evaluation

In situations where the seizure focus is difficult to localize or where results are discordant, Phase II testing via intracranial EEG monitoring is recommended. This can be accomplished by either stereotactic electrocorticography (sEEG) depth electrode placement or subdural electrocorticography (sdEEG) grid placement for cortical monitoring. While intracranial monitoring implantation has been used since the 1960's, implant technology, as well as their indications, have significantly evolved over the past several decades.

The type of Phase II monitoring used and surgical plan vary by indications, patient specific factors, area of interest to be targeted, and practice pattern. There are several benefits of sEEG when compared to subdural grid/strip placement, the most significant one being the ability to sample large bilateral cortical/subcortical regions without the need for a large craniotomy [21–23]. A representative case of a patient with left temporo-occipital epilepsy, and a history of prior resection, who underwent sEEG placement for seizure localization is depicted in **Figure 1**. The minimally invasive nature of depth electrode placement, anchored in the calvarial bone, querying the areas of interest to better localize seizure onset zone can be appreciated. The large craniotomies used for sdEEG placement can add to morbidity, especially in instances requiring extensive bihemispheric mapping. Another advantage of sEEG placement is the relative ease of placement and removal, as these are typically placed percutaneously via a small burr hole and can be removed percutaneously. The stepwise approach of this evaluation allows the epilepsy team time to review the data to better localize the epileptic foci without maintaining the hardware in place for extended periods of time [22, 23]. This contrasts with sdEEG where explantation of the electrodes requires an additional craniotomy and operation, typically followed by resection of the epileptic region at that time. This can prove difficult in complex cases as it may limit the time allowed for the epilepsy and neurosurgical team to review the data and formulate a plan for resection.

While there are several advantages in favor of sEEG, it is not always the most optimal invasive monitoring strategy. In patients who are less than 3 years of age, the

	Evaluation	Function	Strength/Weakness
Phase I			
	Clinical exam	Describe semiology, triggers, and frequency of seizures. Evaluate for neurological deficits	Clinician dependent. Can be difficult to localize lesions.
	Neuropsychology/ neuropsychiatry	Determine subtle neurological/psychological deficits and determine cognitive reserve	Evaluation can be clinician dependent. Standardized forms and help reduce bias and improve interpretability.
	MRI	High-resolution images that can aid in the localization of epileptic pathologies	Able to detect various cerebral pathologies. Can be difficult to interpret subtle abnormalities. Long sequences can require general sedation in the pediatric population.
	fMRI	Determine regions of eloquent cortex	Can help map language, motor, and memory function. Similar reliability to WADA testing. Dependent on patient cooperation.
	MEG	Able to localize epileptic regions based on induction of magnetic fields	Increased sensitivity to cortical epileptic areas. Skull attenuation can limit detection fo deeper lesions.
	Interictal positron emission tomography (PET)	Detection of epileptic foci glucose hypometabolism	Able to detec MRI-negative lesions Glucose hypometabolism is wider than epileptic focus.
	Ictal photon emission CT	Detection of increased cerebral blood flow in the epileptic region	Efficacy depends on timing of tracer injection and seizure frequency.
	Scalp/video EEG	Detection of interictal cortical electrical activity with associated semiology	Inexpensive. Effective in detecting cortical epileptic discharges. Low spatial resolution, skull can cause attenuation of signal.
Phase II			
	Stereo-EEG	Localization of deep cortical epileptic zones when unable to be adequately identified on imaging or scalp EEG	Able to sample bi-hemispheric cortical and subcortical regions simultaneously. Percutaneous placement in the OR and can be removed without the need of additional surgery. No optimal for patients with thin skulls. Lack fidelity with functional cortical mapping.
	Subdural-EEG	Subdural electrode grids/stripes are placed to map cortical function and epileptic regions	High number of electrodes allow for good spatial resolution and functional mapping. Craniotomy needed for placement and removal.

Table 1.
Epilepsy surgery preoperative evaluations.

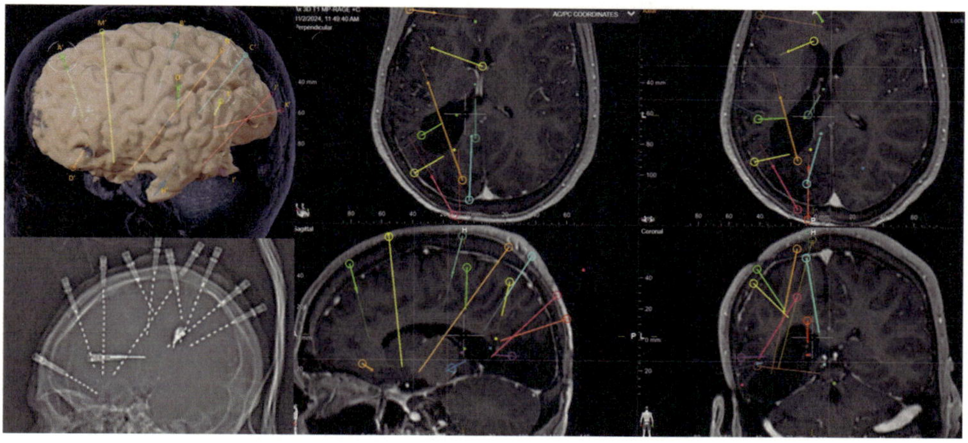

Figure 1.
Stereotactic electroencephalography demonstrative case. The figure above depicts a representative case of a 20-year-old with drug resistant epilepsy, previously treated with a left craniotomy for resection of the temporo-occipital lobes. The patient's phase I data suggested left sided lateralization. sEEG was planned using the patient's preoperative MRI, CT angiogram, and stereotactic planning software completed. On the day of surgery, sEEG was completed using robot assisted techniques and intraoperative CT, querying the left side around the margins of the prior resection as well as the orbitofrontal region, insula, cingulate, and parietal lobe to better localize seizures to the mesial posterior cingulate cortex and gliotic area around the prior resection to guide next steps with therapeutic resective surgery.

thickness of the skull limits the feasibility of percutaneous electrode placement, while sdEEG electrodes can be placed with relatively low complications [24, 25]. Subdural grids and strips are also more favorable in cases where functional mapping is needed as sdEEG have a higher density of cortical contacts compared to sEEG allowing for better spatial resolution [21]. Additionally, the contiguous nature of the sdEEG electrodes allow for improved delineation of the epileptic region compared to normal cerebrum, potentially improving cortical resection without the need interpolation methods used in cases of sEEG placement [22].

Complications following intracranial EEG monitoring are relatively rare, with several meta-analyzes looking at both sEEG and sdEEG electrode placement and the prevalence postoperative hematomas, cerebrospinal fluid (CSF) leak, and infection. In one study assessing sEEG, overall pooled complications were low at 1.3%, with the most common complications being hemorrhage (prevalence of 1.0%) and infection (prevalence of 0.8%) [26]. In sdEEG placement, pooled complications were significantly greater including those for hemorrhage (prevalence 4.0%) and infection (prevalence 3.0%) [25, 27]. Within both groups, rates of morbidity, including permanent neurological deficit, and mortality were similar accounting for only ~0.5% of cases, most of which were related to intracranial hemorrhage [25, 26, 28, 29].

3. Epilepsy surgery

Once the Phase I and/or Phase II workup has been completed and the epileptogenic foci or generalized network is localized, surgical planning can begin, encompassing a wide array of operative techniques and approaches. The therapeutic surgery selected depends greatly on the etiology of the seizures as well as the location of the epileptic zone, so appropriate patient selection is paramount to achieving operative

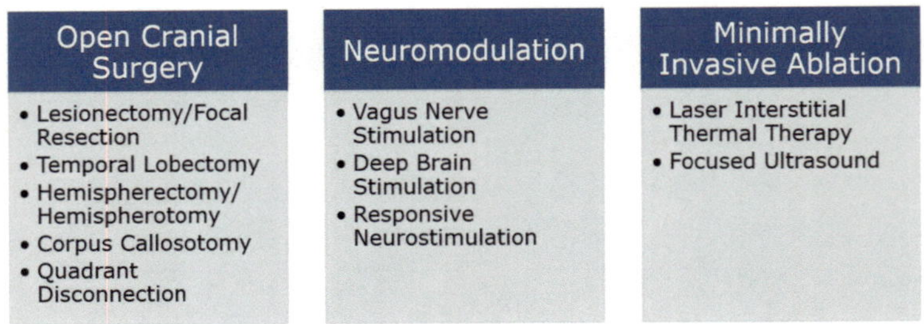

Figure 2.
Types of epilepsy surgery. The figure above depicts the broad categories of epilepsy surgery, including open cranial surgery, neuromodulation, and minimally invasive surgery.

success. Surgery includes open cranial approaches, neuromodulation, and minimally invasive ablation approaches (**Figure 2**). **Table 2** represents a summary of surgical approaches and considerations in the management of epilepsy.

For many of these surgical interventions, surgical adjuncts are paramount. Stereotactic neuronavigation can be used to register the patient's face to their pre-operative magnetic resonance imaging to guide surgical approach and/or resection. Intraoperative ultrasound can be used for real-time dynamic evaluation of neuro-anatomy. Intraoperative CT scan can be used to register surgical robots for stereotactic depth electrode placement. Intraoperative MRI, in centers where it is available, can be used to evaluate extent of resection or provide real-time thermography in cases of laser ablation. These surgical imaging adjuncts, when paired with innovative tools, such as endoscopy, neuromodulation, and ablative procedures, can provide adaptive, state-of-the-art approaches to surgical treatment.

3.1 Lesional resection

In patients who have extra-temporal epileptic lesions, originating from focal cortical dysplasia, tumors, or vascular malformation, most can achieve favorable seizure control upon resection of the offending lesion. Tumors, for example, have been shown to be responsible for 10–30% of DRE with the most common ones being low-grade astrocytomas and gangliogliomas [30]. **Figure 3** depicts focal resection of a tumor via craniotomy. Several studies have demonstrated the efficacy of lesionectomy for seizure control, however, the durability for seizure freedom following resection can vary widely depending on the type of cortical dysplasia, incomplete resection, and longer epilepsy duration, all associated with worse long-term outcomes following surgical intervention [31, 32]. One study demonstrated Engel class I seizure control in 63.2% of patient following surgical resection of non-mesial temporal sclerosis lesions at a mean of 2.9 ± 2.1 years post-operatively [33]. While another study assessing focal cortical dysplasia in pediatric patients demonstrated that 62% of patients achieved Engel class I seizure control at 2 years postoperatively before dropping down to 58% at 5 years [34]. In patients with posterior cortical epileptic foci, seizure freedom was found to be 73.1% within the first 6 months and 54.8% at 6 years demonstrating a lack of durability in some patients [35]. The location of the epileptic foci can also affect the response to surgery, with lesions located in the parietal cortex having worse seizure freedom at 5 years (52%) compared to lesions within the occipital (89%) and parieto-occipital (93%) lobes [35]. Surgical resection of these lesions can be augmented with cortical mapping and electrocorticography (ECoG) to improve resection of the

DOI: http://dx.doi.org/10.5772/intechopen.1012003

Surgery	Indications	Considerations	Outcomes
Lesional/focal resection	Identified structural lesion as the source of epileptic activity (i.e. focal cortical dysplasia, tumors, or vascular malformation)	Ideal for single lesion epilepsy that can be identified on MRI. Multifocal lesional epilepsy can be difficult to treat. Cortical mapping can improve gross total resection and limit damage to normal parenchyma.	Potentially curative if lesion is completely resected.
Temporal lobectomy/ amygdalohippocampectomy	Epileptic zone originating from the temporal lobe (i.e. mesial temporal sclerosis)	Resection of the dominant temporal lobe increases the chances of language, fluency, memory, and visual deficits. fMRI and neuropsychiatric testing can be helpful in preoperative risk assessment. ECoG can assist surgeons in determining the extent of hippocampal resection for prognostication postoperatively.	Have demonstrated seizure freedom between 58 and 81% in the pediatric population.
Hemispherectomy/ hemispherotomy	Epileptic activity that is related to diffuse hemispheric injury either from acquired (i.e. infarction or hemorrhage) or progressive sources (i.e. Rasmussen's encephalitis, Sturge–Weber syndrome)	Multiple surgical approaches may accomplish this disconnection, including vertical and lateral approaches. Anatomic hemispherectomy has fallen out of favor in most cases for functional disconnection surgery given adverse effects (hemosiderosis, hydrocephalus, blood loss). Minimal access or endoscopic techniques allow for smaller incisions and less removal of cortical tissue	Studies have demonstrated 65–90% rates of seizure-freedom on long-term follow-up.
Corpus callosotomy	Allows for hemispheric disconnection and improvement of seizures from infantile spasms/West syndrome, Lennox–Gastaut syndrome (LGS), drop attacks	Complete callosotomy can lead to increased rates of disconnection syndrome compared to anterior callosotomy alone, though complete callosotomy has higher rates of seizure freedom from drop attacks.	Seizure improvement can range from 39 to 90% depending on semiology.
Vagus nerve stimulation (VNS)	Vagal nerve afferent fibers release norepinephrine causing a reduction in seizure frequency via the forebrain, limibic system, and spinal cord	Side effects may include laryngeal motor dysfunction/ paresthesia, bradycardia/heart block, and gastrointestinal distress typically from vagal efferent fibers.	Generally cited as a ~ 50% in seizure reduction in 50% of patients.
Responsive neurostimulation (RNS)	A closed loop system that inhibits epileptic propagation in patients with medically refractory partial seizures and ≤ 2 epileptic foci, broadly being applied to thalamic targets for more generalized types of epilepsy	Currently not FDA approved for pediatric patients with epilepsy; often used off-label. Allows for cortical as well as deep subcortical targeting of multiple thalamic nuclei and the hippocampi involved in epilepsy networks. Expanding indications in diffuse and generalized epilepsy. May limit ability for MRI in the future.	Mostly palliative treatment of DRE with 50–75% seizure reduction and few patients demonstrating seizure freedom.

Surgery	Indications	Considerations	Outcomes
Deep brain stimulation (DBS)	An open loop system that inhibits epileptic propagation in patients with medically refractory seizures	Currently not FDA approved for pediatric patients with epilepsy; often used off-label. Allows for deep subcortical targeting of multiple thalamic nuclei involved in epilepsy networks. May limit ability for MRI in the future.	Mostly palliative treatment of DRE with ~50% in seizure reduction.
Laser interstitial thermal therapy (LITT)	Small/focal lesions (hypothalamic hamartoma, selective amygdalohippocampectomies, etc) that are amenable to thermal ablation. Also used in minimally invasive disconnection surgery via multiple lasers and trajectories.	Minimally invasive procedure that can reach deep subcortical lesions or be used to minimally invasively achieve disconnections. Repeat ablations in iterative strategies are well tolerated. Costs are per laser fiber, which are one-time use.	Seizure control rates between 40 and 60%. Considered to have less longevity than open approaches.
Focused ultrasound (FUS)	Uses high-frequency ultrasound to cause thermal ablation of epileptic lesions.	Currently not FDA approved for epilepsy. Targeting is currently not suitable for superficial lesions. Hair shaving is necessary.	Destructive procedure without surgical incision. Limited studies have demonstrated a reduction in seizure threshold in some but not all patients.

Table 2.
Epilepsy surgery types.

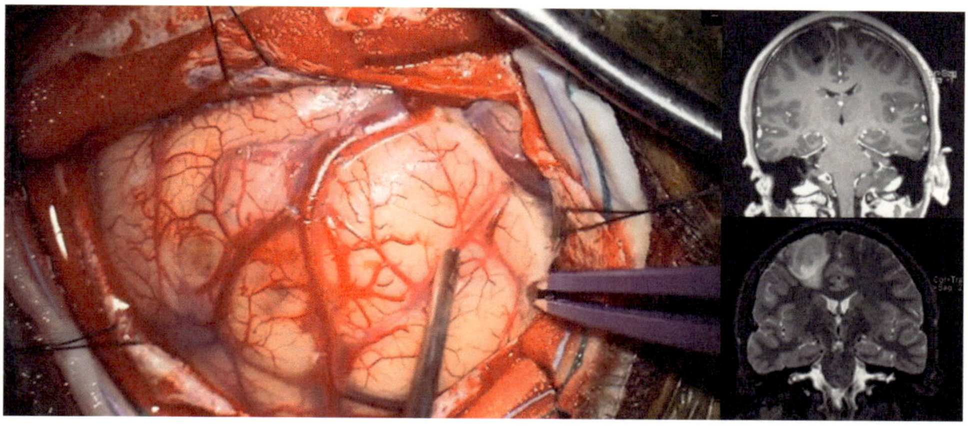

Figure 3.
Demonstrative case of a focal resection of a brain tumor. This 15-year-old patient presented with new onset seizures. They were started on antiseizure medications and MRI demonstrated a T1 hypointense and T2 hyperintense lesion in the right frontal lobe. They underwent gross total resection of the lesion which was tolerated well with resolution of seizure activity; the image depicted above demonstrates the pale, expanded gyrus of the involved lesion. A corticectomy around the lesion was made to dissect the planes of the lesion for resection. Pathology was consistent with astrocytoma WHO grade 3.

epileptic foci and surrounding pathologic tissue while sparing healthy parenchyma thus minimizing neurological impairment [33].

There are risks to every surgery, with open resection, the risks include bleeding, infection, CSF leak, wound healing issues, neurological deficit which varies depending on the location of the craniotomy and region of brain involved, seizure, stroke, coma, and death. While these risks are rare, they are important to discuss with patients in the process of obtaining informed consent to proceed with surgery.

3.2 Temporal lobectomy

The prevalence of temporal lobe epilepsy (TLE) can range from 4 to 10 cases per 1000 in the developed world, frequently caused by mesial temporal sclerosis or imaging negative syndromes such as autosomal dominant TLE, familial (polygenic) TLE, and idiopathic partial epilepsy [36, 37]. Historically there have been two dominant surgical approaches to address temporal epilepsy; anterior temporal lobectomy (ATL) and selective amygdalohippocampectomy (SAH). Typically, ATL is performed by resecting 4–6 cm of the temporal lobe on the non-dominant side and 3.5–4 cm on the dominant side to preserve language and memory function. Selective amygdalohippocampectomy allows for sparing of the lateral temporal lobe and neocortex while removal of the mesial temporal structures and seizure foci is performed (**Figure 4**) [37].

Several studies have demonstrated the advantage of ATL compared to medical management in pediatric patients with DRE related to TLE. Radhakrishnan et al. found that 80.6% of patients were seizure-free at a mean follow-up of 8.1 years, while a randomized trial by Wiebe et al. found that 58% of patients were seizure-free at one-year follow-up [38, 39]. Depending on the pathology and location of epileptic activity, either of the two surgical approaches can be employed by the surgeon, however, there have been several studies that have demonstrated improved seizure control following ATL compared to SAH in the pediatric population, likely related the

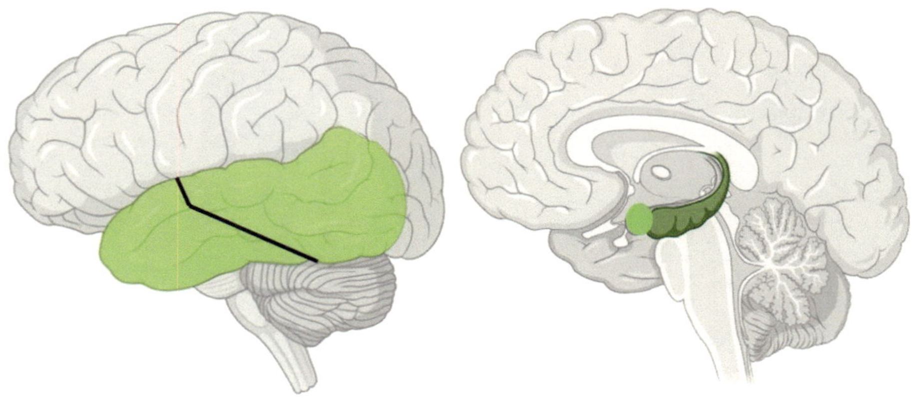

Figure 4.
Anterior temporal lobectomy lateral resection and mesial temporal structures. The figure above shows the lateral resection and mesial structures resected in a standard anterior temporal lobectomy.

increased frequency of pathologies occurring outside of the hippocampus [40, 41]. While intraoperative ECoG can assist surgeons in determining the extent of posterior resection of the hippocampus, possibly sparing functional components, it does not necessarily improve seizure free outcomes compared to anatomical resection [42, 43]. Temporal lobe resection, especially of the dominant lobe, can lead to a number of impairments in language, fluency, memory, and visual deficits [44, 45]. Extensive neuropsychiatric testing and functional MRI can be used to understand the patient's baseline cognitive, language, memory, and functional speech to help optimize safety of resection and perioperative risk stratification. It is not uncommon for speech therapy and/or occupational therapy to be recommended for enhanced postoperative recovery in the weeks to months after surgery for patients with dominant temporal lobe epilepsy who undergo ATL.

3.3 Hemispherectomy

Conditions characterized by diffuse unihemispheric cerebral injury either from an acquired (perinatal infarction, cerebral hemorrhage, hemiconvulsion-hemiplegia epilepsy syndrome, or hemispheric cortical dysplasia) or progressive (Rasmussen's encephalitis, Sturge–Weber syndrome) etiology require a more extensive disconnection of epileptic network [46]. The goal of hemispherectomy or hemispherotomy is to isolate the involved epileptic hemisphere from the rest of the cerebrum, thus preventing the abnormal discharges from propagating throughout the brain. The first anatomical hemispherectomies were conducted by Walter Dandy during resection of large gliomas, involving ligation of the anterior and middle cerebral arteries followed by en bloc resection of the hemisphere [47]. It's uses in epilepsy surgery became popularized in the 1950s to treat infantile hemiplegia [47]. However, by the mid-1960s, significant delayed postoperative complications following anatomical hemispherectomies such as hydrocephalus, subdural fluid collections, and superficial cortical hemosiderosis were noted [48]. Given the morbidity associated with anatomical hemispherectomies, variations began to develop with less emphasis on resection and more on disconnecting the epileptic hemisphere from the healthy one [49–51]. The goals of these functional hemispherectomies were the same as in an anatomical disconnection: disconnection of the cortico-thalamic tract, resection of the mesial

DOI: http://dx.doi.org/10.5772/intechopen.1012003

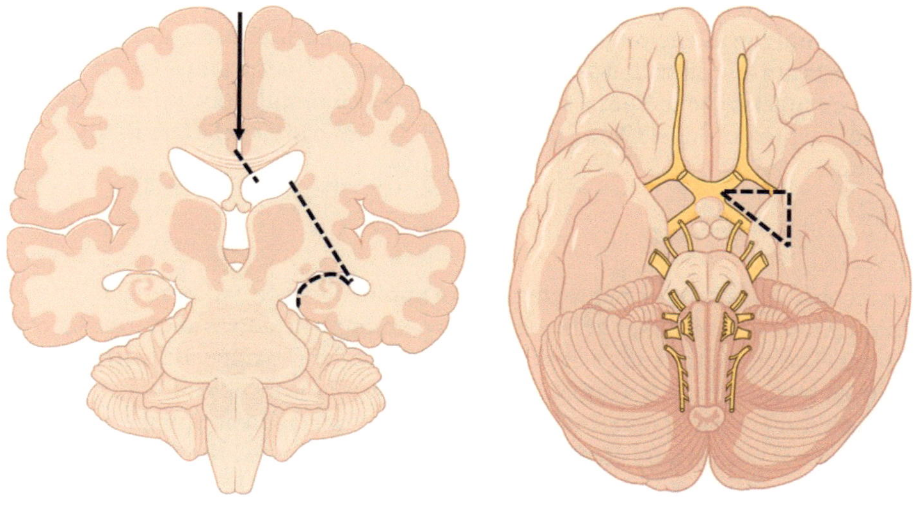

Figure 5.
Hemispheric disconnections via a vertical hemispherotomy. The figure demonstrates the cuts for a vertical hemispherectomy, starting with an interhemispheric approach to a corpus callosotomy, insular disconnection from the lateral aspect of the caudate to the temporal horn for disconnection of the corticothalamic tracts, and mesial temporal disconnection (coronal view). The figure additionally demonstrates the frontobasal disconnection (axial view), depicted with the traditional disconnection using anatomical landmarks of the ACAs, to the ICAs, to the MCA, to the temporal horn (right angle dashed line), vs. the Kawai modification along the optic radiations (oblique dashed line).

temporal structures, corpus callosotomy, and disconnection of the orbito-fronto-hypothalamic tract, all while leaving the diseased brain vascularized and intact (**Figure 5**) [52].

3.4 Hemispherotomy

Hemispherotomy represents progression of the functional hemispherectomy with the major difference being less removal of cortical tissue, however, major disconnection goals remain the same. There are a variety of hemispherotomies that have been described over the years based on surgical approach and order of operations. The peri-insular hemispherotomy consists of several disconnections made through a lateral approach, centered around the circular sulcus, that include transection of the corona radiata, intraventricular callosotomy, posterior hippocampotomy, fronto-basal disconnection, temporal lobe resection, and insular disconnection [53]. This allows for unihemispheric disconnection of epileptic regions from transmitting signals to the contralateral hemisphere, reducing seizure potential. The vertical parasagittal hemispherotomy is another approach allowing for disconnection through an interhemispheric window [49, 54], beginning with an interhemispheric corpus callosotomy, entering the ventricle, allowing for the corona radiata disconnection via the internal capsule before progressing to the trigone of the temporal horn, allowing for disconnection of the temporal lobe, and finally the fronto-basal region is disconnected just anterior to the basal ganglia [49]. Different modifications to these techniques have allowed surgeons to access the various white matter tracts through different approaches based on the specific needs of the surgeon and patient. Another adaptation includes the transsylvian transventricular approach, sought to improve operative times and blood loss [55]. This approach starts with a small craniotomy over the sylvian fissure and transcortical exposure of the lateral ventricle exposing the frontal to the temporal horns encircling the insular cortex. The frontobasal and mesial white matter tracts are disconnected via corpus callosotomy while an amygdalohippocampectomy completes the temporal disconnection. At 46 months postoperatively, 88% of patients achieved Engel Class I outcomes while, 6% had Engel Class III and Class IV outcomes [55].

3.4.1 Endoscopic approaches

As technology continues to progress, more minimally invasive disconnection techniques have emerged that utilize smaller operating corridors while reducing complications. The use of the endoscope in a transventricular disconnection surgery was introduced by Bahuleyan et al. in 2010 [56]. This technique involved placing burr holes at Kocher's and Frazier's point to allow access to the frontal and occipital horns of the lateral ventricle respectively. Rigid endoscopes are then inserted through the burr holes and incised dura with the steps for disconnection accomplished through both openings. The anterior burr hole allows for disconnection of the frontbasal tracts, anterior callosotomy, and unroofing of the anterior temporal horn; while the posterior burr hole provides disconnections to the fornix, posterior callosotomy, and unroofing of the posterior temporal horn [56]. Lam et al. adapted this endoscopic approach in children [57]; their approach used a small paramedian craniotomy in a similar fashion to an interhermispheric approach with a backup temporal incision marked in case the surgery required additional views to complete the frontobasal and insular disconnections. Once the endoscope was inserted and relevant anatomical landmarks identified, the steps toward complete disconnection were performed. Specifically, the corpus callosum was disconnected from rostrum to splenium, the corona radiata (including internal capsule) and frontobasal fibers (uncinate, occipitofrontal fasciculi) were subsequently disconnected via the temporal horn, followed by disconnection of the mesial temporal structures (hippocampus and fornix) to complete the hemispherotomy. A recent case report by LoPresti et al. also describes the use of an endoscopic-assisted posterior quadrantectomy technique in a 17-year-old patient with intractable epilepsy and right hemiparesis secondary to prior CNS lymphoma and treatment [58]. Examining the evolution of endoscopic techniques, appropriate patient selection was paramount in allowing for efficacy and safety of the operation with several authors suggesting that patients with ventriculomegaly and cortical atrophy being optimal candidates to visualize the ventricles and surrounding structures. Additionally, many authors have noted the steep learning curve for these procedures given the novel equipment and surgical approach necessary to perform a successful surgery. Benefits of these procedure may involve decreased intraoperative blood loss, decreased risk of hydrocephalus, improved pain control, and shorter operative times thus improving patient satisfaction and outcomes. Risks may include the standard risks of a craniotomy and the potential risk of recurrent seizures should complete disconnection not be accomplished.

3.5 Corpus callosotomy

Corpus callosotomy is a useful tool for the treatment of a number of pediatric epileptic disorders including infantile spasms/West syndrome, Lennox–Gastaut syndrome (LGS), drop attacks, and severe epilepsy with multiple independent spike foci (SE-MISF) [59, 60]. The procedure essentially disconnects the epileptogenic hemisphere from the normal hemisphere to mitigate seizure propagation. The first corpus

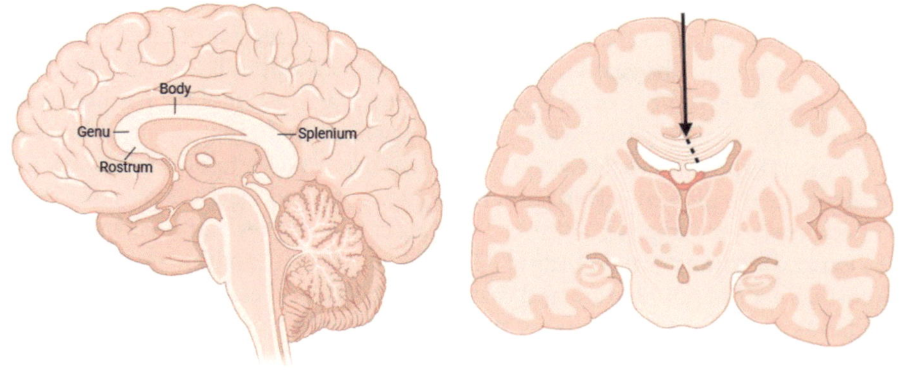

Figure 6.
Corpus callostomy. A corpus callosotomy entails sectioning the corpus callosum along its width, from the rostrum ventrally and anteriorly, to the genu, through the body, to the posterior one third, for an anterior 2/3 corpus callosotomy. For a complete callosotomy, this is extended through the splenium for a complete disconnection.

callosotomy was performed by William P. Van Wagenen in 1939 at the University of Rochester [61]. The procedure was largely abandoned until Roger Sperry published the role of the corpus callosum in interhemispheric connectivity in split-brain studies in the 1950s and 60s [60]. As corpus callosotomies became more widely used to treat intractable epilepsy, studies described disconnection syndrome with a complete callosotomy, thus limitations of the callosotomy to the anterior two-thirds of the corpus callosum were favored for the improved side effect profile. At present, corpus callosotomy represents an effective and well tolerated intervention in pediatric patients with DRE. Both Rathore et al. and Shimuzu demonstrated an improvement in generalized seizure outcomes following both complete and anterior callosotomy, with a ≥ 90% and ~ 87% reduction respectively in each study [62, 63]. Drop attacks specifically were found to benefit from callosal lesioning, with two separate studies demonstrating a ≥ 90% reduction in the severity and frequency of these seizure events [64, 65]. A systemic review conducted by Graham et al. further demonstrated the efficacy of corpus callosotomy in the reduction of drop attacks (67.4%) compared to generalized seizures (39.5%) [66]. Regarding risks of surgery, rates of disconnection syndrome were greater in the complete callosotomy group (12.5%) compared to the anterior callosotomy group (0%), however, there were no differences between surgical or other neurological complications [66]. Disconnection syndrome may result in aphasia and apraxia, with difficulty coordinating movement, and impairment of language and motor function. Thus, patient selection is key to ensure tolerable risk profile and treatment of the seizure types most commonly improved with callosotomy. As such, the use of corpus callostomy remains an integral part in the surgical treatment of DRE and it has become especially useful in the treatment of drop attacks and hemispheric disconnection surgeries (**Figure 6**).

3.6 Laser interstitial thermal therapy

MRI-guided laser interstitial thermal therapy (MRgLITT) has emerged as an exciting tool for the treatment of DRE, especially within the pediatric population. MRgLITT utilizes an optical fiber that is heated by an insulated diode laser, while the catheter is cooled with either saline or CO2 [67]. This laser produces an intense heat that dissipates around the catheter tip, heating the surrounding tissue resulting in thermal denaturation of cellular enzymes and eventually apoptosis. The diode and catheter are advanced into the brain via a stereotactic frame or robot with the target preset by the surgeon. The main advantage to MRgLITT is that it a minimally invasive way to reach deep subcortical regions, making it an ideal tool for patients with lesional (i.e. hypothalamic hamartomas) epilepsy in deep, harder to access locations by conventional approaches. However, it has also been shown to be efficacious for minimally invasive disconnection surgeries as well, applied via multiple laser fibers and trajectories to accomplish MRgLITT corpus callosotomies and hemispherotomies.

The expanding literature on MRgLITT has shown that it can be a vital intervention in the correct patient population, and that it is both safe and efficacious. In a case series of 17 patients (mean age 15.3 years) with DRE and primarily lesional type epilepsy treated with MRgLITT, 41% and 6% of patients achieved Engle I and Engle II outcomes respectively at a mean follow-up of 16.1 months [68]. Four complications were encountered in this series related to inaccurate probe placement, system malfunction, or postoperative dexamethasone induced gastritis. Another small case series of five pediatric patients demonstrated similar results with Engle I outcomes seen in three of the five patients at a maximum of 13 months post-intervention with no complications encountered [69]. To date, medial temporal sclerosis remains the best studied epileptic pathology in MRgLITT (**Figure** 7). While the majority of these studies are in the adult literature, this procedure is applied in children can improve epilepsy outcomes in the pediatric population. Drane et al. assessed the differences in facial recognition and seizure outcomes of MRgLITT and traditional temporal lobectomy in adults with temporal lobe epilepsy [70]. They demonstrated that patients undergoing MRgLITT had improved accuracy on facial recognition with similar rates of seizure control between the two cohhorts, 57.9% treated with MRgLITT and 61.5% who underwent craniotomy. While the use of MRgLITT has some significant benefits in the treatment of select pathologies and patients, gaps still remain in our understanding of this technology and how to best apply it in a clinical setting. Additionally, the long-term outcomes in relation to the treatment of DRE and its durability remain to be seen and will help clinicians and patients to choose the most appropriate therapy for them.

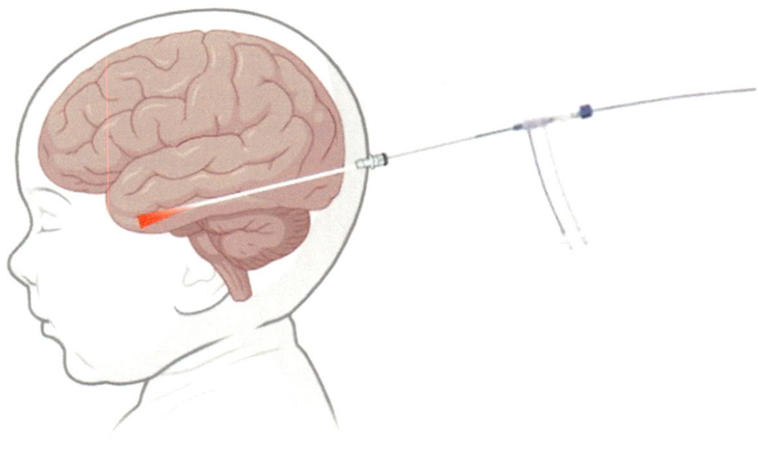

Figure 7.
MRI-guided laser interstitial thermal therapy. This diagram depicts the surgical procedure of MRgLITT, entailing a small burr hole through which an anchor bolt is placed and a laser fiber is passed to the targeted depth stereotactically. This laser fiber is then used to ablate tissue at the target. Its position can be advanced or withdraw along the stereotactic trajectory, which is often targeted along the long-axis of the desired ablation zone.

DOI: http://dx.doi.org/10.5772/intechopen.1012003

3.7 Neuromodulation

While DRE only represents a small subset of epileptic pediatric patients, there can be several factors that can preclude their consideration from resective intervention. Patients without a lesional focus as a clear anatomical cause of their seizures can be difficult to manage even with disconnective surgeries as the epileptic zone might not localize to one hemisphere or location, unfavorable anatomy can limit the operative corridors, or the surgical risk might outweigh the perceived benefits from a larger intervention [19]. In these scenarios, electrical neuromodulation can play a pivotal role in reducing seizure frequency and improving the quality of life in these patients. In 1886, Victor Horsley first utilized electrical cortical stimulation to aid in the resection epileptic foci; while Wilder Penfield expanded this work by mapping our cortical networks to better explain the role of neuroanatomy in seizure development [71], it was not until the 1970s when therapeutic interventions with electrical stimulation began to be used for treatment of epilepsy [72, 73].

3.7.1 Vagus nerve stimulation

In 1990, Penry et al. published results on intermittent vagus nerve stimulation (VNS) for the treatment of intractable seizures [74]. The VNS device consists of an implantable impulse generator that connects to a platinum coated electrode wrapped around the left vagus nerve, delivering an electrical signal in a fashion similar to a cardiac pacemaker (**Figure 8**). While the mechanism of action of vagus nerve stimulators (VNS) on seizure reduction was initially difficult to explain, over the past several decades the interactions between various subcortical areas and the neurotransmitters released by them have shed light on this complex system. At present,

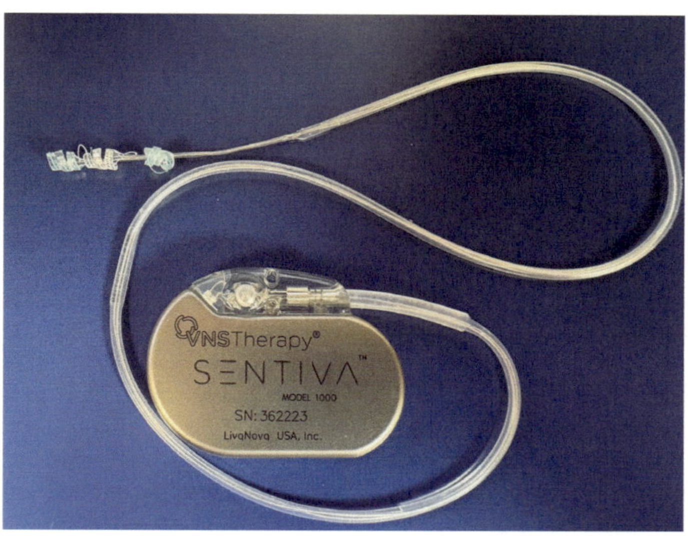

Figure 8.
Vagus nerve stimulator. The vagus nerve stimulator (VNS) consists of an internal pulse generator (IPG) which is placed in a subcutaneous pocket beneath the clavicle and a lead which is connected to the IPG and tunneled to the neck where its three coils, including an anode, anchor, and cathode, are implanted around the vagus nerve, within the carotid sheath. These are performed on the left side to minimize risk of cardiac arrhythmia, associated with vagus nerve function on the right side. Other risks of surgery include bleeding, infection, hoarseness of voice, dysphagia, pain, vocal fold paralysis, risk of damage to surrounding structures, and failure to control seizures.

the hypothesis is that vagal nerve afferents synapsing on the nucleus of the solitary tract (NST), with projections to the locus coeruleus (LC) and dorsa raphe, increase noradrenergic tone in the CNS via norepinephrine release into the forebrain, limbic system, and spinal cord thus reducing seizure activation and propagation [75]. While these afferent fibers are thought to mediate the antiseizure benefits of VNS placement, vagus nerve efferents cause many of the side effects associated with their use including laryngeal motor dysfunction/paresthesia, bradycardia/heart block, and gastrointestinal distress [75].

In 1997, the FDA approved VNS implantation in children >12 years of age with medically intractable partial seizures who are not candidates for surgical resection. Twenty years later, the FDA modified its approval to include pediatric patients ≥4 years of age, thus expanding its application to many more individuals. Since its introduction, there have been a number of studies delineating the efficacy and optimal patient selection for this form of intervention. In 2013, the American Association of Neurology (AAN) issued an update on their guidelines for VNS placement citing several studies demonstrating a > 50% in seizure reduction in 55% of pediatric patients survey across 13 different studies, with a pooled seizure freedom rate of 7% [76]. Patients with Lennox–Gastaut syndrome can be particularly difficult to treat, but also demonstrated a similar responder rate of 55% and a > 50% reduction in seizure frequency [76]. A more recent systemic review by Hajtovic et al. attempted to better isolate genetic conditions that had more robust benefits following VNS implantation. Their study found that patients with tuberous sclerosis had a pooled seizure freedom rate of 40%, with 31% of patients experiencing a ≥ 90% seizure reduction rate, and 68% of patient with a ≥ 50% reduction. Other etiologies such as Dravet syndrome, Rett syndrome, and various epileptic genetic disorders had limited efficacy based their small sample sizes and limited studies available for interpretation [77]. Given the heterogeneity in response rates and seizure freedom following VNS implantation, more research is needed to better identify patients who will have greater benefits following treatment. In light of this, institutions both in the US and Canada are collaborating with the Connectomic Profiling and Vagus Nerve Stimulation Outcomes Study (CONNECTiVOS) to identify patient biomarkers that can be used to select the ideal patient for VNS intervention [78].

3.7.2 Responsive neurostimulation

The role of neuromodulation in epilepsy was further expanded in 2013 with the introduction of responsive neurostimulation (RNS), a closed-loop implantable pulse generator with two electrodes that detect a seizure and deliver targeted therapy to the epileptic source [75]. The RNS system exerts is antiseizure effects through electrical disruption of the seizure focus and inhibits the propagation of electrical signals to distal cortical regions [75]. Additional underlying mechanisms could also include disruption of axonal conduction from high-frequency stimulation and as well as changes in synaptic plasticity and neurogenesis from chronic stimulation [75]. In RNS, an implanted device sits within the skull and is connected to two electrodes, targeted either subcortically or cortically, to sense and stimulate in response to seizures (**Figure 9B**). A demonstrative case treated with RNS is depicted in **Figure 10**.

At present, RNS is approved for patients ≥18 years of age with medically refractory partial seizures and ≤ 2 epileptic foci [11]. While not currently FDA approved in the pediatric population, there are ongoing efforts to expand its application and off-label use to include pediatric patients who suffer from DRE, focusing increasing

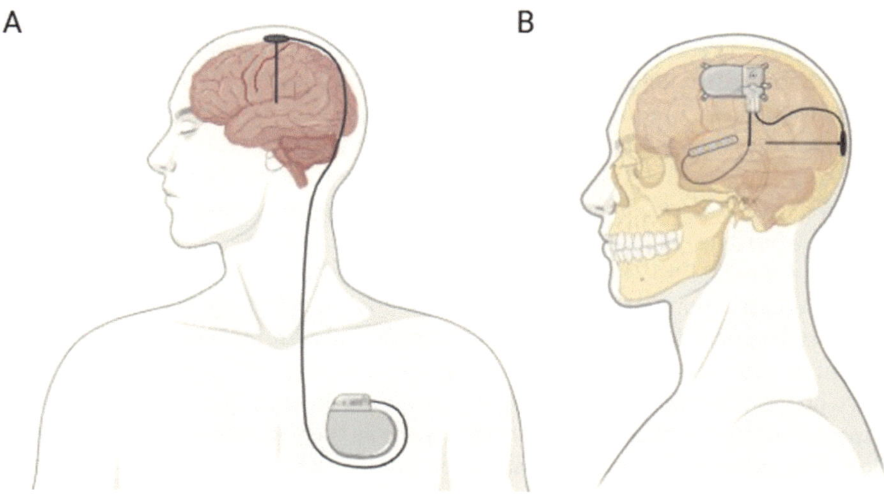

Figure 9.
Deep brain stimulation and responsive neurostimulation. Diagram A depicts the surgical approach to deep brain stimulation (DBS) where one to two depth electrodes are placed stereotactically, through burr holes, anchored to the skull, and tunneled with lead extenders to an internal pulse generator (IPG) subcutaneously on the chest wall which stimulates networks involved in seizures to interrupt seizure activity. Diagram B depicts the surgical approach to responsive neurostimulation (RNS) where an implanted device sits within the skull and is connected to two electrodes, targeted either subcortically or cortically, to sense and stimulate in response to seizures.

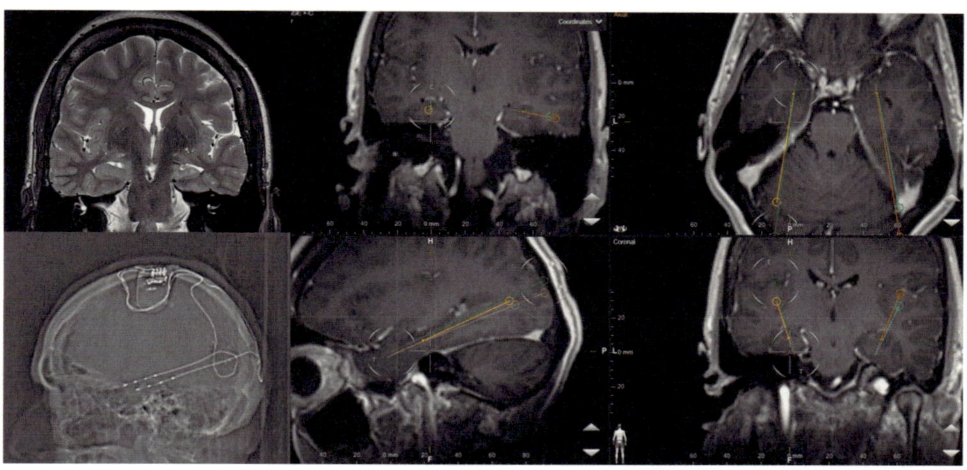

Figure 10.
Demonstrative case of a RNS for bitemporal epilepsy. The patient had a history of bitemporal epilepsy. MRI demonstrated T2/FLAIR signal in the left hippocampus, consistent with mesial temporal sclerosis. Phase I evaluation was consistent with bitemporal epilepsy. They underwent bihippocampal RNS placement for treatment of epilepsy with reduction in seizure burden and frequency.

efforts on generalized or diffuse etiologies via thalamic stimulation. A recent pediatric case study demonstrated that RNS implantation can be a safe and effective treatment with improvement of seizure control in a 16-year-old female with incomplete resection of focal cortical dysplasia and continued debilitating seizures despite antiseizure medication management [79]. A separate study assessed the safety of RNS implantation in an off-label study of 27 pediatric patients (ages 7–17 years) demonstrating an overall reduction in seizure frequency with >50% of the patients have an improvement of 75% or more in seizure frequency at an average follow-up period of 22 months [80]. A recent literature review and case series also demonstrated improvement in seizure reduction following centromedian nucleus of the thalamus (CMT) RNS implantation in 21 adult patients and three pediatric cases [81]. The authors demonstrated an average seizure reduction of 77% with 95% and 55% of adult patients experiencing a > 50% and ≥ 90% reduction in seizure frequency respectively. In their pediatric subset, all patients experienced between a 70–100% improvement in their seizure burden.

There are several limitations that make placement of an RNS system more challenging in the pediatric population compared to their adult counterparts. For one, the pulse generator is designed to be placed in full-thickness calvariums which can limit their placement in patients with thinner and/or growing skulls. Additionally, for small, deep thalamic nuclei with precise targeting, it is unknown how the growing pediatric skull may impact depth electrode placement over time as the patient ages and continues to develop. Furthermore, MRI is currently contraindicated in patients with RNS implantation which will limit future neuroimaging in pediatric patients. Lastly, the RNS system has demonstrated mostly palliative seizure control with few patients become completely seizure-free over time, impacting seizure frequency and severity and significant rates, but not often providing cure [79]. Risks of RNS placement include bleeding, infection, failure to control seizures, damage to surrounding structures, neurological deficits, seizure, stroke, coma, and death. Despite this, a preeminent open-label prospective clinical trial (RESPONSE study) is currently under investigation assessing the safety and efficacy of RNS implantation for patients between the ages of 12–17 years old with the first patient treated in May of 2022 [82, 83].

3.7.3 Deep brain stimulation

The application of electrical stimulation to cortical and subcortical regions for the treatment of neurological disorders has existed for over 70 years [84]. These electrical impulses are thought to inactivate the implanted structure via high-frequency stimulation causing time locking of the natural axonal activity [75]. Initially used in the treatment of movement disorders [84, 85], DBS has been well documented as an effective and safe surgery, with its application in the treatment of epilepsy is evolving. In the 1980s, the Irving Cooper placed electrodes within the anterior nucleus of the thalamus (ANT) and cerebellum for the treatment of intractable partial seizures with clinical and pharmacologic improvement in the patient's semiology [86]. Since then, a number of targets have been proposed as potential targets in the treatment of epilepsy including the cerebellum, thalamus, hippocampus, caudate, nucleus accumbens, and subthalamic nucleus, among others [87].

Thalamic DBS for DRE has been FDA approved since 2018. Surgery entails the placement of two depth electrodes stereotactically, through burr holes, anchored to the skull, and tunneled with lead extenders to an internal pulse generator (IPG) subcutaneously on the chest wall which stimulates networks involved in seizures to interrupt seizure activity (**Figure 9A**). Risks of DBS include bleeding, infection, failure to control seizures, damage to surrounding structures, neurological deficits, seizure, stroke, coma, and death.

The best reported and most efficacious DBS targets for epilepsy are in the thalamus, specifically the anterior nucleus of the thalamus (ANT), centromedian nucleus of the thalamus (CMT), dorsalis medialis (DM) nucleus, and pulvinar nucleus [87]. The ANT has significant connectivity throughout the mesial/anterior frontal lobe and temporal lobes, areas often associated with epileptic foci [54, 88]. In 2010, a multicenter study assessing bilateral ANT DBS lead placement demonstrated a seizure reduction of at least 50% in 56% of adult patients treated at 2 years compared to the control group with 14 patients being seizure free at 6-months [89]. The Stimulation of the Anterior Nucleus of the Thalamus for Epilepsy (SANTÉ) study published seven-year follow-up data demonstrating robust long-term seizure control with a median seizure reduction of 75% and an overall patient mortality of 6.9 deaths per 1000 person-years [90].

While the ANT has demonstrated the best efficacy for focal seizures, CMT has emerged as a target of interest for generalized and multifocal seizures [87]. In epilepsy patients, activation of the CMT exhibits diffuse ipsilateral cortio-cortical evoked potentials, with projections to a number of nuclei including the caudate, lentiform nucleus, sensorimotor/premotor corticies, and subthalamic nucleus among others [91, 92]. The use of the CMT in epilepsy targeting was popularized by Velasco et al. in 1987 in five patients with multifocal/generalized epilepsy [93]. A recent prospective open-label study of 20 patients (median age 15.5 years of age) demonstrated a > 50% in seizure reduction in 90% of their patients with one patient being seizure free at 2 years [94] . In 2022, Dalic et al. reported their results of 20 patients with Lennox–Gastaut syndrome and CMT DBS implantation, demonstrating a 53.8% reduction in seizure frequency compared to the control group, however, this was not statistically significant [95].

As with the prior two thalamic nuclei, both the DM and pulvinar remain areas of investigation for DRE treatment. Stimulation of the DM shows activation of the ipsilateral orbitofrontal, mesial/lateral frontal area, along with some activation of the mesial temporal region [91]. The pulvinar represents the largest thalamic nucleus with a number of connections to both cortical and subcortical regions. The medial pulvinar specifically has projections to typical epileptic areas including the amygdala, hippocampus, temporal neocortex, cingulate and orbitofrontal cortex [96]. There remain limited clinical studies related to seizure control and the DM and pulvinar, with the majority of studies existing in animal models or small cases series. In a study of eight patients with DRE originating from the temporal lobe and pulvinar DBS, five of the eight patients experiencing less severe seizures with improved levels of consciousness compared to those patients with non-pulvinar stimulation [97].

While much of the DBS literature has examined adults. Several case reports and retrospective series detail safety and efficacy in children with epilepsy. There are ongoing clinical trials in North America examining the role of DBS in pediatric epilepsy.

4. Future directions

The treatment of DRE remains a challenging and often multi-factorial discussion between the patient and the treating clinicians, including epileptologists, neuropsychologists, and neurosurgeons. This pathology can prove to be even more complicated in pediatric patients given their growing anatomy, limited working space, diverse pathologies, and developing brain impacted by the side effects of sedating seizure medication and unrelenting seizures. It is therefore imperative that a thorough workup be conducted for all patients presenting for seizure evaluation so that the semiology can be described and etiologies localized. The use of both Phase I and Phase II testing allows the clinical team to proceed in an organized fashion so that a complete evaluation is conducted for each evaluation. Based on this workup, referral for epilepsy surgery is recommended. As our understanding of epilepsy continues to evolve and the treatment options become more diverse, the goal is for future interventions to be tailored to individuals based on their seizures and pathology. At the heart of the presurgical evaluation is the multidisciplinary care coordination between the epilepsy neurology and neurosurgical team.

At present, surgical resection remains a mainstay in the treatment of DRE, especially in patients with localizable disease during testing. However, neuromodulation allow neurosurgeons to operate on previously untreatable patients and minimally invasive approaches to surgery allow neurosurgeons to provide surgical treatment with fewer adverse effects while improving seizure outcomes. In patients who are not candidates for either resection or disconnection surgeries, newer palliative options such as MRgLITT, VNS, RNS, and DBS are becoming more accessible and expanding the indications for intervention. Furthermore, adaptation of existing technologies, like stereotactic radiosurgery, which are not commonly used for the treatment of epilepsy, have a role in the treatment of epilepsy related to deep, hard to reach lesions such as hypothalamic hamartomas. While these interventions are further defining their place in the treatment paradigm for DRE, new technologies are already in development offering less invasive approaches.

4.1 Focused ultrasound

Focused ultrasound (FUS) is a promising new therapy that already has FDA approval for the treatment of essential tremor and Parkinson's disease. FUS entails a high-frequency ultrasound beam amplified and localized to a focal target within the brain, typically with the assistance of MR imaging, causing acoustic ablation of the target [98]. The application of FUS in epilepsy remains limited and an area of future interest given its non-invasive nature and ease of operation. Several case series out of Asia have demonstrated its efficacy in lowering seizure thresholds in some but not all patients with limited adverse effects [99–101]. However, in these studies, the sample sizes are small with minimal long-term follow-up over 12 months, making their generalizability limited.

While there is still significant research needed to address the current shortcomings of these newer technologies, they remain viable options for many patients. Larger clinical trials with a more pediatric focus are also needed to help refine the selection criteria and report the outcomes for this under-researched population. Additionally, long-term follow-up comparing approaches and outcomes will help elucidate who may benefit most from which procedure going forward when there is overlap in what may be offered.

5. Conclusion

Epilepsy is a common, life-changing condition. When medical management fails, surgical treatment is recommended to, where able provide seizure freedom, and improve seizure burden, reduce seizure frequency, improve quality of life, and improve changes of long-term survival. We summarize updates in epilepsy surgery evaluation and provide a comprehensive review of the current status of pediatric epilepsy surgery, including advances and innovations in the field. Pediatric DRE is a highly complex pathology that continue to push the boundaries of both neurology

DOI: http://dx.doi.org/10.5772/intechopen.1012003

and neurosurgery; ongoing innovations in technology and diagnostic and/or therapeutic approaches continue to advance the field.

Conflicts of interest

Sandi Lam discloses research funding from:

PCORI: Comparative effectiveness of palliative surgery versus additional antiseizure medications for Lennox–Gastaut Syndrome.

PCORI supplement: Indirect costs of care for families of patients with Lennox–Gastaut Syndrome.

NIH/NINDS SBIR: Assessment of CSF Shunt Flow with Thermal Anisotropy Measurement Device.

NSF SBIR II: Development of a Noninvasive, Wireless Telemedicine Flow Sensor for Patients with Hydrocephalus.

Northwestern Institute of Global Health: Building Capacity for Treatment of Surgical Epilepsy in Uganda.

Sandi Lam discloses Industry and No- Profit COI:

Livanova: Advisory Board.

Synergia: Advisory Board.

BrainLab: Consultant.

Encoded Therapeutics: Consultant.

Jaguar Therapeutics: Consultant and Chair of DSMB.

Ovid Therapeutics: Consultant.

Brain Recovery Project/Pediatric Epilepsy Surgery Alliance: Board Member.

CURE Epilepsy: Scientific Board Member.

Author details

Ryan Kelly[1], Melissa A. LoPresti[2*] and Sandi Lam[3]

1 Department of Neurosurgery, Rush Medical Center, Chicago, IL, USA

2 Department of Neurosurgery, Rochester University Medical Center, Rochester, NY, USA

3 Division of Pediatric Neurosurgery, Lurie Children's Hospital, Northwestern University, Chicago, IL, USA

*Address all correspondence to: mlopresti01@gmail.com

References

[1] Fiest KM, Sauro KM, Wiebe S, Patten SB, Kwon CS, Dykeman J, et al. Prevalence and incidence of epilepsy: A systematic review and meta-analysis of international studies. Neurology. 2017;**88**(3):296-303

[2] Guerrini R. Epilepsy in children. Lancet. 2006;**367**(9509):499-524

[3] Aaberg KM, Gunnes N, Bakken IJ, Lund Søraas C, Berntsen A, Magnus P, et al. Incidence and prevalence of childhood epilepsy: A nationwide cohort study. Pediatrics. 2017;**139**(5):e20163908

[4] Asarnow RF, LoPresti C, Guthrie D, Elliott T, Cynn V, Shields WD, et al. Developmental outcomes in children receiving resection surgery for medically intractable infantile spasms. Developmental Medicine and Child Neurology. 1997;**39**(7):430-440

[5] Jonas R, Nguyen S, Hu B, Asarnow RF, LoPresti C, Curtiss S, et al. Cerebral hemispherectomy: Hospital course, seizure, developmental, language, and motor outcomes. Neurology. 2004;**62**(10):1712-1721

[6] Schnier C, Chin RF. Mortality in children with epilepsy: Cohort study using the clinical practice research datalink. Seizure. 2023;**109**:77-82. DOI: 10.1016/j.seizure.2023.05.020. Epub 2023 May 30

[7] Berg AT, Nickels K, Wirrell EC, Geerts AT, Callenbach PM, Arts WF, et al. Mortality risks in new-onset childhood epilepsy. Pediatrics. 2013;**132**(1):124-131. DOI: 10.1542/peds.2012-3998. Epub 2013 Jun 10

[8] Kløvgaard M, Lynge TH, Tsiropoulos I, Uldall PV, Banner J, Winkel BG, et al. Epilepsy-related mortality in children and young adults in Denmark: A nationwide cohort study. Neurology. 2022;**98**(3):e213-e224. DOI: 10.1212/WNL.0000000000013068. Epub 2021 Nov 18

[9] Berg AT, Shinnar S, Testa FM, Levy SR, Smith SN, Beckerman B. Mortality in childhood-onset epilepsy. Archives of Pediatrics & Adolescent Medicine. 2004;**158**(12):1147-1152. DOI: 10.1001/archpedi.158.12.1147

[10] Gadgil N, LoPresti MA, Muir M, Treiber JM, Prablek M, Karas PJ, et al. An update on pediatric surgical epilepsy: Part I. Surgical Neurology International. 2019;**10**:257

[11] Karsy M, Guan J, Ducis K, Bollo RJ. Emerging surgical therapies in the treatment of pediatric epilepsy. Translational Pediatrics. 2016;**5**(2):67-78

[12] Tang F, Hartz AMS, Bauer B. Drug-resistant epilepsy: Multiple hypotheses, few answers. Frontiers in Neurology. 2017;**8**:301

[13] Zhang L, Hall M, Lam SK. Comparison of long-term survival with continued medical therapy, vagus nerve stimulation, and cranial epilepsy surgery in paediatric patients with drug-resistant epilepsy in the USA: An observational cohort study. The Lancet Child & Adolescent Health. 2023;**7**(7):455-462. DOI: 10.1016/S2352-4642(23)00082-2. Epub 2023 Jun 2

[14] Ali R, Connolly ID, Feroze AH, Awad AJ, Choudhri OA, Grant GA. Epilepsy: A disruptive force in history. World Neurosurgery. 2016;**90**:685-690

[15] Kwan P, Arzimanoglou A, Berg AT, Brodie MJ, Allen Hauser W,

Mathern G, et al. Definition of drug resistant epilepsy: Consensus proposal by the ad hoc Task Force of the ILAE Commission on therapeutic strategies. Epilepsia. 2010;**51**(6):1069-1077

[16] Jette N, Reid AY, Wiebe S. Surgical management of epilepsy. CMAJ. 2014;**186**(13):997-1004

[17] Beier AD, Rutka JT. Hemispherectomy: Historical review and recent technical advances. Neurosurgical Focus. 2013;**34**(6):E11

[18] Jehi L, Jette N, Kwon CS, Josephson CB, Burneo JG, Cendes F, et al. Timing of referral to evaluate for epilepsy surgery: Expert consensus recommendations from the Surgical Therapies Commission of the International League against Epilepsy. Epilepsia. 2022;**63**(10):2491-2506. DOI: 10.1111/epi.17350. Epub 2022 Jul 17

[19] Ryvlin P, Cross JH, Rheims S. Epilepsy surgery in children and adults. Lancet Neurology. 2014;**13**(11):1114-1126

[20] Engel J. Why is there still doubt to cut it out? Epilepsy Currents. 2013;**13**(5):198-204

[21] Jayakar P, Gotman J, Harvey AS, Palmini A, Tassi L, Schomer D, et al. Diagnostic utility of invasive EEG for epilepsy surgery: Indications, modalities, and techniques. Epilepsia. 2016;**57**(11):1735-1747

[22] Kovac S, Vakharia VN, Scott C, Diehl B. Invasive epilepsy surgery evaluation. Seizure. 2017;**44**:125-136

[23] Iida K, Otsubo H. Stereo-electroencephalography: Indication and efficacy. Neurologia Medico-Chirurgica (Tokyo). 2017;**57**(8):375-385

[24] Taussig D, Dorfmüller G, Fohlen M, Jalin C, Bulteau C, Ferrand-Sorbets S, et al. Invasive explorations in children younger than 3 years. Seizure. 2012;**21**(8):631-638

[25] Arya R, Mangano FT, Horn PS, Holland KD, Rose DF, Glauser TA. Adverse events related to extraoperative invasive EEG monitoring with subdural grid electrodes: A systematic review and meta-analysis. Epilepsia. 2013;**54**(5):828-839

[26] Mullin JP, Shriver M, Alomar S, Najm I, Bulacio J, Chauvel P, et al. Is SEEG safe? A systematic review and meta-analysis of stereo-electroencephalography-related complications. Epilepsia. 2016;**57**(3):386-401

[27] Dorfmüller G, Ferrand-Sorbets S, Fohlen M, Bulteau C, Archambaud F, Delalande O, et al. Outcome of surgery in children with focal cortical dysplasia younger than 5 years explored by stereo-electroencephalography. Child's Nervous System. 2014;**30**(11):1875-1883

[28] Hamer HM, Morris HH, Mascha EJ, Karafa MT, Bingaman WE, Bej MD, et al. Complications of invasive video-EEG monitoring with subdural grid electrodes. Neurology. 2002;**58**(1):97-103

[29] Serletis D, Bulacio J, Bingaman W, Najm I, González-Martínez J. The stereotactic approach for mapping epileptic networks: A prospective study of 200 patients. Journal of Neurosurgery. 2014;**121**(5):1239-1246

[30] Bauer R, Dobesberger J, Unterhofer C, Unterberger I, Walser G, Bauer G, et al. Outcome of adult patients with temporal lobe tumours and medically refractory focal epilepsy. Acta Neurochirurgica. 2007;**149**(12):1211-1217

[31] Simasathien T, Vadera S, Najm I, Gupta A, Bingaman W, Jehi L. Improved outcomes with earlier surgery for

intractable frontal lobe epilepsy. Annals of Neurology. 2013;**73**(5):646-654

[32] McIntosh AM, Averill CA, Kalnins RM, Mitchell LA, Fabinyi GCA, Jackson GD, et al. Long-term seizure outcome and risk factors for recurrence after extratemporal epilepsy surgery. Epilepsia. 2012;**53**(6):970-978

[33] Dhiman V, Rao S, Sinha S, Arimappamagan A, Mahadevan A, Bharath RD, et al. Outcome of lesionectomy in medically refractory epilepsy due to non-mesial temporal sclerosis (non-MTS) lesions. Clinical Neurology and Neurosurgery. 2013;**115**(12):2445-2453

[34] Choi SA, Kim SY, Kim H, Kim WJ, Kim H, Hwang H, et al. Surgical outcome and predictive factors of epilepsy surgery in pediatric isolated focal cortical dysplasia. Epilepsy Research. 2018;**139**:54-59

[35] Jehi LE, O'Dwyer R, Najm I, Alexopoulos A, Bingaman W. A longitudinal study of surgical outcome and its determinants following posterior cortex epilepsy surgery. Epilepsia. 2009;**50**(9):2040-2052

[36] Téllez-Zenteno JF, Hernández-Ronquillo L. A review of the epidemiology of temporal lobe epilepsy. Epilepsy Research and Treatment. 2012;**2012**:630853

[37] Nickels KC, Wong-Kisiel LC, Moseley BD, Wirrell EC. Temporal lobe epilepsy in children. Epilepsy Research and Treatment. 2012;**2012**:849540

[38] Wiebe S, Blume WT, Girvin JP, Eliasziw M. A randomized, controlled trial of surgery for temporal-lobe epilepsy. The New England Journal of Medicine. 2001;**345**(5):311-318

[39] Radhakrishnan A, Menon R, Abraham M, Vilanilam G, Sharma S, Thomas B, et al. Predictors of outcome after surgery in 134 children with drug-resistant TLE. Epilepsy Research. 2018;**139**:150-156

[40] Josephson CB, Dykeman J, Fiest KM, Liu X, Sadler RM, Jette N, et al. Systematic review and meta-analysis of standard vs selective temporal lobe epilepsy surgery. Neurology. 2013;**80**(18):1669-1676

[41] Datta A, Sinclair DB, Wheatley M, Jurasek L, Snyder T, Quigley D, et al. Selective amygdalohippocampectomy: Surgical outcome in children versus adults. The Canadian Journal of Neurological Sciences. 2009;**36**(2):187-191

[42] McKhann GM, Schoenfeld-McNeill J, Born DE, Haglund MM, Ojemann GA. Intraoperative hippocampal electrocorticography to predict the extent of hippocampal resection in temporal lobe epilepsy surgery. Journal of Neurosurgery. 2000;**93**(1):44-52

[43] Schwartz TH, Bazil CW, Walczak TS, Chan S, Pedley TA, Goodman RR. The predictive value of intraoperative electrocorticography in resections for limbic epilepsy associated with mesial temporal sclerosis. Neurosurgery. 1997;**40**(2):302-311

[44] Yam D, Nicolle D, Steven DA, Lee D, Hess T, Burneo JG. Visual field deficits following anterior temporal lobectomy: Long-term follow-up and prognostic implications. Epilepsia. 2010;**51**(6):1018-1023

[45] Lassonde M, Sauerwein HC, Jambaqué I, Smith ML, Helmstaedter C. Neuropsychology of childhood epilepsy: Pre- and postsurgical assessment. Epileptic Disorders. 2000;**2**(1):3-13

[46] Young CC, Williams JR, Feroze AH, McGrath M, Ravanpay AC, Ellenbogen RG, et al. Pediatric functional hemispherectomy: Operative techniques and complication avoidance. Neurosurgical Focus. 2020;**48**(4):E9

[47] Kim J, Park E, Shim K, Kim DS. Hemispherotomy and functional hemispherectomy: Indications and outcomes. Journal of Epilepsy Research. 2018;**8**(1):1-5

[48] Oppenheimer DR, Griffith HB. Persistent intracranial bleeding as a complication of hemispherectomy. Journal of Neurology, Neurosurgery, and Psychiatry. 1966;**29**(3):229-240

[49] Delalande O, Bulteau C, Dellatolas G, Fohlen M, Jalin C, Buret V, et al. Vertical parasagittal hemispherotomy: Surgical procedures and clinical long-term outcomes in a population of 83 children. Neurosurgery. 2007;**60**(2 Suppl. 1):ONS19-32; discussion ONS32

[50] Rasmussen T. Hemispherectomy for seizures revisited. The Canadian Journal of Neurological Sciences. 1983;**10**(2):71-78

[51] Ignelzi RJ, Bucy PC. Cerebral hemidecortication in the treatment of infantile cerebral hemiatrophy. The Journal of Nervous and Mental Disease. 1968;**147**(1):14-30

[52] Morino M, Shimizu H, Ohata K, Tanaka K, Hara M. Anatomical analysis of different hemispherotomy procedures based on dissection of cadaveric brains. Journal of Neurosurgery. 2002;**97**(2):423-431

[53] Villemure J, Daniel RT. Peri-insular hemispherotomy in paediatric epilepsy. Child's Nervous System. 2006;**22**(8):967-981

[54] Keller SS, O'Muircheartaigh J, Traynor C, Towgood K, Barker GJ, Richardson MP. Thalamotemporal impairment in temporal lobe epilepsy: A combined MRI analysis of structure, integrity, and connectivity. Epilepsia. 2014;**55**(2):306-315

[55] Schramm J, Kral T, Clusmann H. Transsylvian keyhole functional hemispherectomy. Neurosurgery. 2001;**49**(4):891-901

[56] Bahuleyan B, Manjila S, Robinson S, Cohen AR. Minimally invasive endoscopic transventricular hemispherotomy for medically intractable epilepsy: A new approach and cadaveric demonstration. Journal of Neurosurgery. Pediatrics. 2010;**6**(6):536-540

[57] Wagner K, Vaz-Guimaraes F, Camstra K, Lam S. Endoscope-assisted hemispherotomy: Translation of technique from cadaveric anatomical feasibility study to clinical implementation. Journal of Neurosurgery. Pediatrics. 2018;**23**(2):178-186

[58] LoPresti MA, Wagner K, Lam S. Endoscope-assisted posterior quadrant disconnection plus corpus callosotomy: Case report. Journal of Neurosurgery. Pediatrics. 2021;**27**(4):406-410

[59] Wong T, Kwan S, Chang K, Hsiu-Mei W, Yang T, Chen Y, et al. Corpus callosotomy in children. Child's Nervous System. 2006;**22**(8):999-1011

[60] Vaddiparti A, Huang R, Blihar D, Du Plessis M, Montalbano MJ, Tubbs RS, et al. The evolution of corpus callosotomy for epilepsy management. World Neurosurgery. 2021;**145**:455-461

[61] Mathews MS, Linskey ME, Binder DK, William P. Van Wagenen and the first corpus callosotomies for

epilepsy. Journal of Neurosurgery. 2008;**108**(3):608-613

[62] Shimizu H. Our experience with pediatric epilepsy surgery focusing on corpus callosotomy and hemispherotomy. Epilepsia. 2005;**46**(Suppl. 1):30-31

[63] Rathore C, Abraham M, Rao RM, George A, Sankara Sarma P, Radhakrishnan K. Outcome after corpus callosotomy in children with injurious drop attacks and severe mental retardation. Brain & Development. 2007;**29**(9):577-585

[64] Cendes F, Ragazzo PC, da Costa V, Martins LF. Corpus callosotomy in treatment of medically resistant epilepsy: Preliminary results in a pediatric population. Epilepsia. 1993;**34**(5):910-917

[65] Pinard JM, Delalande O, Chiron C, Soufflet C, Plouin P, Kim Y, et al. Callosotomy for epilepsy after West syndrome. Epilepsia. 1999;**40**(12):1727-1734

[66] Graham D, Tisdall MM, Gill D. Corpus callosotomy outcomes in pediatric patients: A systematic review. Epilepsia. 2016;**57**(7):1053-1068

[67] Missios S, Bekelis K, Barnett GH. Renaissance of laser interstitial thermal ablation. Neurosurgical Focus. 2015;**38**(3):E13

[68] Lewis EC, Weil AG, Duchowny M, Bhatia S, Ragheb J, Miller I. MR-guided laser interstitial thermal therapy for pediatric drug-resistant lesional epilepsy. Epilepsia. 2015;**56**(10):1590-1598

[69] Curry DJ, Gowda A, McNichols RJ, Wilfong AA. MR-guided stereotactic laser ablation of epileptogenic foci in children. Epilepsy & Behavior. 2012;**24**(4):408-414

[70] Drane DL, Loring DW, Voets NL, Price M, Ojemann JG, Willie JT, et al. Better object recognition and naming outcome with MRI-guided stereotactic laser amygdalohippocampotomy for temporal lobe epilepsy. Epilepsia. 2015;**56**(1):101-113

[71] Feindel W. The contributions of Wilder Penfield to the functional anatomy of the human brain. Human Neurobiology. 1982;**1**(4):231-234

[72] Cooper IS, Amin I, Gilman S. The effect of chronic cerebellar stimulation upon epilepsy in man. Transactions of the American Neurological Association. 1973;**98**:192-196

[73] Van Buren JM, Wood JH, Oakley J, Hambrecht F. Preliminary evaluation of cerebellar stimulation by double-blind stimulation and biological criteria in the treatment of epilepsy. Journal of Neurosurgery. 1978;**48**(3):407-416

[74] Penry JK, Dean JC. Prevention of intractable partial seizures by intermittent vagal stimulation in humans: Preliminary results. Epilepsia. 1990;**31**(Suppl 2):40

[75] Wong S, Mani R, Danish S. Comparison and selection of current implantable anti-epileptic devices. Neurotherapeutics. 2019;**16**(2):369-380

[76] Morris GL, Gloss D, Buchhalter J, Mack KJ, Nickels K, Harden C. Evidence-based guideline update: Vagus nerve stimulation for the treatment of epilepsy: Report of the Guideline Development Subcommittee of the American Academy of Neurology. Neurology. 2013;**81**(16):1453-1459

[77] Hajtovic S, LoPresti MA, Zhang L, Katlowitz KA, Kizek DJ, Lam S. The role of vagus nerve stimulation in genetic etiologies of drug-resistant epilepsy: A

meta-analysis. Journal of Neurosurgery. Pediatrics. 2022;**29**(6):667-680

[78] Siegel L, Yan H, Warsi N, Wong S, Suresh H, Weil AG, et al. Connectomic profiling and vagus nerve stimulation outcomes study (CONNECTiVOS): A prospective observational protocol to identify biomarkers of seizure response in children and youth. BMJ Open. 2022;**12**(4):e055886

[79] Singhal NS, Numis AL, Lee MB, Chang EF, Sullivan JE, Auguste KI, et al. Responsive neurostimulation for treatment of pediatric drug-resistant epilepsy. Epilepsy & Behavior Case Reports. 2018;**10**:21-24

[80] Panov F, Ganaha S, Haskell J, Fields M, La Vega-Talbott M, Wolf S, et al. Safety of responsive neurostimulation in pediatric patients with medically refractory epilepsy. Journal of Neurosurgery. Pediatrics. 2020;**26**(5):525-532

[81] Vessell M, Willett A, Chapman B, Bina R, Ball T, Mutchnick I, et al. Evidence for thalamic responsive neurostimulation in treatment of adult and pediatric epilepsy. Stereotactic and Functional Neurosurgery. 2023;**101**(2):75-85

[82] RNS® System Responsive Stimulation for Adolescents with Epilepsy Study. 2022 November 11

[83] Meglio M. First Patient Treated in Adolescent Epilepsy Trial Assessing NeuroPace RNS System. 2022. Available from: https://www.neurologylive.com/view/first-patient-treated-adolescent-epilepsy-trial-assessing-neuropace-rns-system [Accessed: April 29, 2023]

[84] Delgado JMR, Hamlin H, Chapman WP. Technique of intracranial electrode implacement for recording and stimulation and its possible therapeutic value in psychotic patients. Confinia Neurologica. 1952;**12**(5-6):315-319

[85] Bekhtereva NP, Grachev KV, Orlova AN, Iatsuksl n. [Utilization of multiple electrodes implanted in the subcortical structure of the human brain for the treatment of hyperkinesis]. Zhurnal Nevropatologii i Psikhiatrii Imeni S.S. Korsakova. 1963;**63**:3-8

[86] Upton AR, Amin I, Garnett S, Springman M, Nahmias C, Cooper IS. Evoked metabolic responses in the limbic-striate system produced by stimulation of anterior thalamic nucleus in man. Pacing and Clinical Electrophysiology. 1987;**10** (1 Pt 2):217-225

[87] Fisher RS. Deep brain stimulation of thalamus for epilepsy. Neurobiology of Disease. 2023;**179**:106045

[88] Warsi NM, Yan H, Suresh H, Wong SM, Arski ON, Gorodetsky C, et al. The anterior and centromedian thalamus: Anatomy, function, and dysfunction in epilepsy. Epilepsy Research. 2022;**182**:106913

[89] Fisher R, Salanova V, Witt T, Worth R, Henry T, Gross R, et al. Electrical stimulation of the anterior nucleus of thalamus for treatment of refractory epilepsy. Epilepsia. 2010;**51**(5):899-908

[90] Salanova V, Sperling MR, Gross RE, Irwin CP, Vollhaber JA, Giftakis JE, et al. The SANTÉ study at 10 years of follow-up: Effectiveness, safety, and sudden unexpected death in epilepsy. Epilepsia. 2021;**62**(6):1306-1317

[91] Zumsteg D, Lozano AM, Wieser HG, Wennberg RA. Cortical activation with deep brain stimulation of the anterior thalamus for epilepsy. Clinical Neurophysiology. 2006;**117**(1):192-207

[92] Ilyas A, Pizarro D, Romeo AK, Riley KO, Pati S. The centromedian nucleus: Anatomy, physiology, and clinical implications. Journal of Clinical Neuroscience. 2019;**63**:1-7

[93] Velasco F, Velasco M, Ogarrio C, Fanghanel G. Electrical stimulation of the centromedian thalamic nucleus in the treatment of convulsive seizures: A preliminary report. Epilepsia. 1987;**28**(4):421-430

[94] Cukiert A, Cukiert CM, Burattini JA, Mariani PP. Seizure outcome during bilateral, continuous, thalamic centromedian nuclei deep brain stimulation in patients with generalized epilepsy: A prospective, open-label study. Seizure. 2020;**81**:304-309

[95] Dalic LJ, Warren AEL, Bulluss KJ, Thevathasan W, Roten A, Churilov L, et al. DBS of thalamic centromedian nucleus for Lennox-Gastaut syndrome (ESTEL trial). Annals of Neurology. 2022;**91**(2):253-267

[96] Benarroch EE. Pulvinar: Associative role in cortical function and clinical correlations. Neurology. 2015;**84**(7):738-747

[97] Filipescu C, Lagarde S, Lambert I, Pizzo F, Trébuchon A, McGonigal A, et al. The effect of medial pulvinar stimulation on temporal lobe seizures. Epilepsia. 2019;**60**(4):e25-e30

[98] Lescrauwaet E, Vonck K, Sprengers M, Raedt R, Klooster D, Carrette E, et al. Recent advances in the use of focused ultrasound as a treatment for epilepsy. Frontiers in Neuroscience. 2022;**16**:886584

[99] Lee CC, Chou CC, Hsiao FJ, Chen YH, Lin CF, Chen CJ, et al. Pilot study of focused ultrasound for drug-resistant epilepsy. Epilepsia. 2022;**63**(1):162-175

[100] Abe K, Yamaguchi T, Hori H, Sumi M, Horisawa S, Taira T, et al. Magnetic resonance-guided focused ultrasound for mesial temporal lobe epilepsy: A case report. BMC Neurology. 2020;**20**(1):160

[101] Yamaguchi T, Hori T, Hori H, Takasaki M, Abe K, Taira T, et al. Magnetic resonance-guided focused ultrasound ablation of hypothalamic hamartoma as a disconnection surgery: A case report. Acta Neurochirurgica. 2020;**162**(10):2513-2517